Living the EnerQi Connection

Living the EnerQi Connection

Manifesting Positive Change
Discover Your Abundant Natural Energy
with the LAINE System

Sheri Laine LAc,
Diplomate of Acupuncture

Health Communications, Inc.
Deerfield Beach, Florida

www.hcibooks.com

Disclaimer: The advice contained in this book is not intended as a substitute for the advice and/or medical care of the reader's physician. The reader should generally consult with a physician in matters relating to his or her health. Any eating or exercise regimen should be undertaken after consulting with the reader's physician.

Library of Congress Cataloging-in-Publication Data
is available through the Library of Congress

© 2014 Sheri Laine

ISBN-13: 978-07573-1819-1 (Paperback)
ISBN-10: 07573-1819-3 (Paperback)
ISBN-13: 978-07573-1820-7 (ePub)
ISBN-10: 07573-1820-7 (ePub)

Publisher: Health Communications, Inc.
        3201 S.W. 15th Street
        Deerfield Beach, FL 33442–8190

Cover art © Fotolia.com
Cover and interior design by Lawna Patterson Oldfield

Contents

Acknowledgments

I have been very fortunate to have met many incredible people through my work who have given me much to think about, grow from, and experience. Through their kindness, trust, and faith, I have become a deeper, richer person and a more skilled practitioner. I am grateful for their confidence in my ability, wisdom, and experience.

What we have all heard is true: Dreams really can and do come true. Another truth is that it does take a village—without mine, I would not be the woman I am today. Many, many thanks to the beautiful, kind, creative, supportive, and generous women and men I am so fortunate to have in my life. Your enduring EnerQi truly empowers and nourishes mine.

To my life partner, Gary Seidler, whose love and support fills me with happiness, laughter, and creativity every day, thank you. Much appreciation and gratitude to Peter Vegso, president of HCI, for taking a chance. Thank you to the HCI family, who have all kindly and generously extended their friendship and trust. A special thank you to my editors, Carol Killman Rosenberg, Erika Burke, and Allison Janse for their support and expert guidance.

To my beloved Chinese grand master, Dr. Richard Teh-Fu Tan—"Kam pi," thank you again for leading me into a deeper understanding of the many mysteries of life, for being there for me no matter what the time or the tide, and for guiding me to the heart and soul of Chinese medicine. *Namaste.*

Preface: How I Got Here

When I reflect on the events of my childhood, I clearly recognize that I was being prepared mentally and spiritually for the role I now play in my life as an Oriental Medicine practitioner. I feel very strongly about using the term "Oriental medicine" instead of "Eastern medicine." Eastern Medicine is the definition of medicine practiced only in China; I discuss and practice Oriental medicine in the broader sense of a complete lifestyle that is practiced all over the Orient. Oriental medicine includes the practice of acupuncture, Chinese herbology, nutrition, gentle exercise and movement, mental harmony, and bodywork. It took me many years to find my career path—and it was a road of synchronicities that led me here.

Growing up in Southern California at the base of the tall foothills in the San Fernando Valley, I lived in a home surrounded by a variety of plants, including flowers, eucalyptus trees, pine trees, and flowering cacti. Behind our backyard, separated by only a fence, was an expansive field where the neighborhood white horse, Diller, and a few mules grazed. I spent a lot of time on the other side of the fence, hanging out with Diller and giving him body rubs. We had a quiet understanding of each other. I knew I was different from most children, and he was more than happy to accept me just the way I was.

My siblings, our neighborhood friends, and I would spend hours outdoors, hiking, exploring, and making forts. Always on the lookout for interesting plants, leaves, flowers, and bark, I would happily pick, gather, and carefully wrap my treasures in a hankie before putting them in my pocket for transport home to my "hospital fort."

My brothers had fitted my hospital fort with a pair of long shelves supported by old red bricks. We found the bricks left over from a neighbor's patio project and liberated thick boards from an old abandoned truck at the top of the next hill, hauling them back together.

I placed old mayonnaise and mustard jars with the labels soaked off onto these shelves and filled them with plants, flowers, and leaves collected from our long, carefree hikes. I put new white labels on the jars that reflected the names of the plants and flowers inside. I made "medicine tea" by mixing a bit of this and a bit of that onto squares of paper towels, which I folded into an envelope, giving medicinal tea bags to my "sick patients" to take home with them.

White sheets and towels that I had stolen from my mother's linen closet were arranged in rows side by side for my patients to lie down on when they would come in for a treatment.

One of my favorite games was Operation. I would practice my doctor skills as often as I could get someone to play with me. I was also proudly in possession of my very own doctor's bag, which included a plastic stethoscope, an otoscope, a thermometer, tongue depressors, and a plastic syringe. My doctor's bag also held several Sucrets metal tins, which I had filled with various sizes of cactus needles that I had painstakingly collected from the many succulent cacti around our home. I would thread the needles through pieces of white gauze to keep them in neat rows according to size.

Once I had convinced the gang (or anyone, for that matter) to come to my hospital fort, I somehow also talked them into lying down and letting me give them "shots" all over their bodies with my odd little assortment of needles. Many neighborhood friends would scramble with real fear in their eyes, running full speed down the hill from my fort at the first sign of my needles. Others would stay and play along.

During this time in my childhood, from about age seven to twelve, when I would lie down in my bed to go to sleep at night, a ticker tape of seemingly random numbers would run through my mind's eye, such as 1, 22, 35, 6, 7, 5, 17, 11, 4, 36. The combinations of numbers mesmerized me. This ticker tape would generally go on for quite some time. I would often repeat the numbers as they came into my head—much like saying a mantra—before falling asleep. I never gave much thought to what they meant, although they were rather comforting.

By the time I was nearly thirteen years old—growing into adolescence, my idyllic childhood behind me—I no longer played in my hospital fort, and my numbers mantra had faded away. I moved on with my life, with its adolescent up and downs. My fascination with my doctor's bag and all that it meant to me was but a distant memory. Eventually, I pursued my teaching degree with the intent of becoming an early-childhood Montessori teacher.

While attending classes in 1979, I gave birth to my beautiful daughter, Amber. Born at home, she was very healthy, and there were no complications. However, at the age of six months, she suffered a skull fracture that led to vision loss in her left eye. My grief was immeasurable. Amber's injury contributed to my decision to learn everything I could about natural medicine to help her as well as to heal myself.

A single mom, I started out training in reflexology while holding down various waitressing jobs. In 1981, my daughter and I were living in San Diego, and I had decided to apply for a position in the office of a highly sought-after natural physician, Dr. Barnet Meltzer. Although Dr. Meltzer did not offer me a position, as I was waiting for my interview I met a woman much like myself with whom I became instant friends. Her friend Bill was studying to become an acupuncturist. Bill needed people to practice on so he could complete his internship and graduate. My new friend recruited me for a treatment.

I was not at all quite sure what a "treatment" meant. However, I was immediately intrigued. When I met Bill at the school's clinic, he came into the treatment room, which had rows of massage tables covered with white sheets. As I looked around, my mind flashed back to the hospital fort of my childhood. He opened a silver tin, revealing needles all lined up by size very neatly on rows of gauze. Again my psyche traveled back, to the cactus needles in the Sucrets tins! I felt the most incredible sense of awareness, familiarity, and awe. In that moment, I knew I had found my next path—or perhaps my path had found me?

The needles did not hurt at all, and while they were in place I felt totally relaxed. I could feel my body vibrating, as if currents of electricity were running up and down my arms and legs. It was an amazing experience. I fell into the most restful sleep, although I remember being aware of the pulsations through my body. My body felt strengthened yet relaxed, and my mind was clear and sharp. I felt high on life for days afterward.

Before we left the clinic, Bill took me to the Chinese herb room where all the herbs were stored in preparation for formulations. They were all lined up on wooden shelves in glass jars with white labels—roots, branches, flowers, and bark. There was a very large roll of white paper in which to wrap the herbs as the formulas were being made. Even though it was decades since my time in the woods as a child, I felt I was once again standing before my "hospital" shelves lined with plant-filled jars. The very thing I had been doing as a child in play was before me now! I knew this was more than a coincidence; I was being given the most amazing opportunity to explore my first passion and devotion.

I enrolled in classes the very next semester. Although it took me a year of attendance at the local community college to fill in some prerequisite premed classes and sciences, I never wavered from my decision to study Oriental medicine—nor did I give a thought to how I was going to pay for my education.

On my first day of class at the California Acupuncture College, which soon became the Pacific College of Oriental Medicine, we studied *point prescription formulations*. These are the potentially hundreds of combinations of acupuncture points that a student must learn and commit to memory in order to pass the state boards.

Point prescriptions are studied to learn how to understand, respond to, and treat the symptoms or syndrome that a patient is experiencing. They are, in essence, the myriad point patterns that one can use to correct the flow of *qi* (pronounced "chee" and sometimes spelled *chi*), which is life force or vital energy. The meridians, the pulsating energy fields that line the body, are all numbered; each number has a corresponding function and interacts with another number and function on another meridian or on its own meridian.

- A point prescription for mania looks like this: Lung 1, Heart 9, Pericardium 9, Large Intestine 1, San Jiao 1, Small Intestine 1—or 1, 9, 9, 1, 1, 1.
- Another example, for abdominal pain, looks like this: Stomach 36, Spleen 4, Ren 10, Spleen 6, Stomach 29, Ren 4—or 36, 4, 10, 6, 29, 4.

There were the numbers again—those numbers that had run like an endless ticker tape through my mind as a child for all those years. I *knew* these combinations; they were already in my consciousness. They felt deeply familiar to me.

Traditionally, Oriental medicine (which falls under the umbrella term *Eastern medicine or Chinese medicine*) was passed down from father to son or from master to apprentice. A Chinese medicine master is a teacher who is usually also a doctor who has been in practice for many years. Masters demonstrate skill, intellect, and infinite wisdom, perfecting their technique and style in diagnosis, formulation, and treatment. They constantly strive for and achieve powerful levels of excellence while earning the respect and admiration of their peers, students, and patients.

When a master chooses a student, the decision is not made lightly, because the relationship and commitment span a lifetime. My Chinese medicine master, Dr. Richard Teh-Fu Tan Tan, chose me carefully to be his apprentice to study Chinese ancestral secrets. We had met in passing ten years earlier at the Pacific College of Oriental Medicine, when Dr. Tan was finishing his internship at the school clinic during my first year. (Although Dr. Tan was a health professional in China, he had to retake his boards in this country and complete another internship). I had been practicing acupuncture in my own private clinic for about four years when Dr. Tan and I unexpectedly ran into each other at a conference a decade after our first meeting. A month later, he invited me to lunch.

Dr. Tan interviewed me over the course of many lunch and dinner meetings, quizzing me intensely on a whole range of topics, including who my patients were, what their symptoms were, what acupuncture points I chose and why, and what my herbal formulation plans and nutritional evaluations were. He wanted to know what their physical and mental responses were and what I planned for my next treatments. It was like an interrogation. He threw out herbal formulations in Chinese and asked me if I would consider using them instead of my intended choices. Of course, some of them were the wrong formulas, and I would have to tell him the right ones—in Chinese!

This interview process took almost a year. Once Dr. Tan had made the decision to take me on as his student, he invited me to his favorite Chinese restaurant for an elaborate fish banquet to celebrate the beginning of our work together. I was honored to be among Dr. Tan's other apprentices, who were all senior to me.

Once Dr. Tan deemed me a serious and deserving student, he opened up and shared with me the most amazing stories, treatment strategies, and "secret" herbal formulations. Some of these treatment strategies came from his own brilliant calculations, whereas others were handed down from generations past—from his great-great grandfather, who was a physician, to many governors in China. Dr. Tan is a no-nonsense teacher. He practices and teaches with a watchful, intuitive gaze. He does not suffer fools lightly, has a wonderful sense of the world, and is trusted by all who know him. He is admired for his wisdom and knowledge.

I have been studying with Dr. Tan for more than seventeen years now. He teaches in both Chinese and English, which initially made it hard to figure out his exact message. For the first year, I was not permitted to ask any questions. My job was simply to observe his treatment techniques, chart patients' progress, clean the rooms, answer the phones, make appointments, and handle payments at the front desk. Although I was doing monotonous and sometimes tedious tasks (think *The Karate Kid*) for much of the first few years, I spent as much time as possible at Dr. Tan's elbow in the treatment rooms and in the herbal pharmacy, watching him treat his patients and prepare the herbal formulations.

In China, doctors often see and treat ten to twenty-five patients together in the same room or down long hall-ways, talking openly about physical maladies without any thought to privacy. (Since China is so heavily populated, the Chinese do not have the same views on privacy or place the same kind of value on privacy that Americans do).

Dr. Tan treats his patients in the United States in a similar way. Understanding his culture, they don't seem to mind. He would often see up to forty-five patients in my one four-hour weekly shift! Watching him in his clinic and listening to how he answers his patients' and students' questions has most certainly made me a wiser doctor and a more ana-lytical thinker. More important, he has consistently showed me what I want and need to know about Oriental medicine.

I've learned so much from Dr. Tan, from my studies, and from the many patients with whom I have worked. I enjoy sharing my knowledge through teaching, speaking profes-sionally, writing articles for periodicals, Internet e-zines, my blog, and social media sites.

I have written *Living the EnerQi Connection* because I have found that most people interested in acupuncture, and Ori-ental medicine in general, have similar questions. Much of the available information on Eastern medicine (another umbrella term for both Oriental and Chinese medicine) is confusing—even to me at times, although I have been practicing for more than twenty-eight years. With the West's heavy reliance on prescription medications and attempts at self-medication, I have found that there is an overwhelming need for Oriental medicine in our society, and this book attempts to bring to light its many benefits.

I also want to share what it means and feels like to be a part of living the EnerQi connection—the energetic vibration we emit that connects us all. With a basic understanding of Oriental medicine and its concepts, as well as with the newfound awareness of your own EnerQi vibration, you too will be on your way to the vibrant health, balance, wellness, and vitality that is your divine right. Whether you are looking to become balanced, to feel better, stay healthy or you are just curious, this book may provide you with the answers you have been looking for.

Introduction:
Enhancing Your EnerQi

Welcome to a better understanding of the concepts of the body's energy and the energy that surrounds us in the world. This knowledge will allow you to better participate in your own living process, healing process, and health maintenance. I use the following simple mnemonic device, which I call the LAINE system, with my patients to illustrate our incredible nature:

Learn (about incredible natural energy)

Align (restore balance)

Inform (use newfound information to integrate lifestyle changes)

1

Natural (discover the health and vitality that is part of your inherent nature)

Energy (harness your internal power)

Reading this book will help you to learn about incredible natural energy and how it can change and enhance your life. It is my sincere wish that by the time you have finished reading, you will be inspired to experience acupuncture, embrace its profound effects, and enjoy a balanced lifestyle.

Do you ever wonder what the word *balance* means in relationship to how we live and behave in our mental, physical, and emotional lives, and why a lot of us seem to be reading and talking about balance more frequently? As a twenty-eight-year practitioner of Oriental medicine, I know that balance always comes up in conversation with my patients, regardless of their sex or age. Oriental medicine is designed to preserve qi energy, the life force that circulates in our bodies and around all of us throughout the day and even when we are at rest or asleep.

Balance is the way in which we maintain harmony and preserve our vital qi force field. EnerQi is the combination of all the factors that bring you to your optimal state of well-being. I have coined the term *EnerQi* (ener-chee) to describe this harmonization and preservation of our inner and outer power.

So how does EnerQi apply to our lives? How can we use it to create more equilibrium and happiness in our lives and within our communities? The chapters that follow will provide you with insight about our natural energy and how you can begin to live a more balanced lifestyle for richer health and deeper happiness.

As you will learn, creating balance in our lives means to sleep deeply and well; to exercise regularly and eat delicious, whole foods that replenish and nourish our bodies; to enjoy art, literature, music, and good conversation with friends while sharing our feelings openly in ways that make others desire to listen and engage with us; to show compassion for ourselves and others; and to go quietly within to develop clear answers to cloudy questions.

In all these ways, we become strong conduits of our own EnerQi vibration. This means being as real and as true to ourselves as we can possibly be, right here today, in this moment. If sadness or loss is prevalent in our lives, we do not pretend it away. We allow ourselves to feel the pain. We have the ability and the courage to look at any situation with as much awareness and honesty as we are capable of in any given moment. Balance is the ability to love others in the ways we want to be loved in return.

Maintaining an attitude of gratitude in life, practicing acceptance and forgiveness, and facing and accepting the challenges we all share with a positive approach will bring us truth and inner happiness. Accessing the EnerQi of the situation, whatever it may be, creates a way to restore or maintain balance. As we move about our lives in our world and in our neighborhoods, we give off an energetic vibration, and others pick up on it. When we are in balance, or on an even keel, a wave of good EnerQi is created. You can choose to begin creating yours now.

PART I

Learn

LEARNING IS WEIGHTLESS,
A TREASURE YOU CAN ALWAYS
CARRY EASILY.

—Chinese proverb

Chapter 1

Understanding EnerQi and How It Works

---

*Believe the best is
yet to come.*

—Anonymous

What's the secret? Why is it that some of us get noticed in life and others feel left behind? Why is it that some people have greater challenges in attaining success or happiness? Could it be that the energetic vibration that surrounds us, or draws others to us, is part of the equation for success and happiness in our lives?

Qi, our life force or vital energy, is an electromagnetic vibration that circulates in and around each of us. This energy system carries our physical, mental, and spiritual power within it, and it is what energetically charges us. Everything carries with it its own qi, its own energetic vibrational force. EnerQi (pronounced *ener-chee*) is the outward vibration, whereas qi is the circulating energy within and outside our bodies.

Look around you. Notice your environment. How does it make you feel? How do you feel when you are in the mountains or by the sea, gazing up at the blue or gray sky and smelling the fresh air that circulates around you? After spending time outside in nature, most of us feel charged, elevated, connected, and changed—in harmony. This feeling of harmony is a result of the energy your body has absorbed from your surroundings.

How do you feel when you walk into a nice home or restaurant? You probably notice that it makes you feel good. Compare that feeling to walking into a dark, dingy, dirty establishment. Most of us can't wait to exit a place with a weird, "ick factor" vibration. It is a relief to be away from it.

When you are in tune with your body, your body is in tune with the environment, which makes you much more sensitive to, and in touch with, other people and your surroundings. Although we interact with a lot of people every day, every so often we feel connected with someone in particular. Have you ever been inexplicably drawn to a complete stranger—be it a member of the same or the opposite sex? When this happens, we feel compelled to talk with that person, he or she interests us. That powerful connection is a result of our energetic vibration. We are attracted to that particular vibration because it connects with and balances our own energy.

Knowing this allows you to stay in tune with your inner and outer vibration, harnessing your EnerQi. By keeping your vibration at its highest frequency, attracting similar vibrations, and, conversely, knowing when to walk away when your vibration does not resonate with another's, you attract vibrant health and well-being.

Yin and Yang: Opposite Energies for Balance

Oriental medicine practitioners use the concept of opposite, interdependent energies to highlight the necessity of balance in the body and in the environment. The warmth of summer surrenders to the coolness of autumn and later to the coldness of winter. The cycle continues as the shorter, colder, darker days give way to spring, with its longer and lighter days, and continues to the warmth of summer. The night always becomes the day, and the day always becomes the night.

Like day and night, yin and yang (pronounced "yawng") are opposites that are intertwined. One always balances the other. They are didactic partners, always connected. Yin is the black, internal, feminine, earth, wet, cool, intuitive, and contemplative energy. Yang is the white, external, masculine, heaven, dry, hot, action-oriented energy.

We all have a unique combination of yin and yang qi in our bodies. This combination can change daily, based on our lifestyle choices. We feel yin energy when we don't want to get out of bed in the morning, and we feel yang energy when we are wide awake, ready to start our day even before the alarm goes off.

We are all born with a certain amount of qi, which is the body's constitutional strength. Think of qi as your body's root system; it is always in place to feed and nourish you, especially if you have taken good care of it. This root strength, qi, can be maintained and strengthened through a balanced lifestyle supported by healing practices, such as acupuncture and herbal remedies. When our qi is in balance, the EnerQi vibration we emit becomes more powerful.

Enhancing Our Qi and EnerQi

Acupuncture and herbal medicines are a powerful way to enhance our qi and our EnerQi. We experience our qi in terms of our energy level. Our qi changes based on how we take care of ourselves and on the lifestyle choices we make. We all know how bad we feel when we're caught off balance and have not been good to ourselves. When we are balanced, our energetic frequency is raised to a much higher level, making us feel stronger and more alive than ever before. The more we focus on the principles of balance in life, the better able and more in touch we will become at fine-tuning our body's EnerQi vibration with ease.

Qi expresses itself as a strong energy field that becomes stronger when we are balanced. By using healthy living and powerful thoughts to balance your qi and thereby enhance your EnerQi, you will feel healthier, happier, more relaxed, and fulfilled. You will also have the enhanced ability to absorb the positive EnerQi vibrations from the world around you. You will find that your body just works better.

You will see the positive magnetic effects of your amplified EnerQi as you become more balanced. People will naturally gravitate to you when your EnerQi is pulsating with health, creativity, and vitality. When you are balanced, you are happy and empowered to lead the life you want, get the job you want, and enjoy the types of relationships you want. These positive aspects of life are attracted to your energetic force field. That is pulsating magnetic qi manifested powerfully.

What is your highest vision for yourself and the life you would like to create? What does it look like to be, to do, and to have positive, powerful experiences in your life? Having balanced EnerQi is relative to the experience of where you choose to place your power and your thoughts. The decision to live in a high EnerQi vibration also has incredible power emotionally and spiritually.

Life happens to us all. We can ride the inevitable waves of change much more profoundly and powerfully when we connect to the force within that allows us to shift our perception. We can all access a physical, mental, and soulful connection to our highest self, to shine our brightest light.

Honestly access the EnerQi in your life. Start by taking the quiz that follows. Accept where you are right now and what your state is, then proceed with a plan to elicit the desired effect for change.

Assessing Your EnerQi Vibration Quiz

If I always do what I've always done,
I'll always get what I've always gotten.

—ANTHONY ROBBINS

LET'S FIND OUT IF YOUR LIFE IS IN BALANCE. Read through the following questions as you think about your life. Choose the answer that most closely reflects what is true for you. When you're finished, count the number of a, b, and c answers. Refer to the key that follows the questions to find out how balanced you are. That's the first step in making any necessary changes for greater health and well-being.

1. When I wake up, I feel:
   a. Refreshed and ready to start my day.
   b. Sluggish, but after some caffeine I'm raring to go.
   c. I'm dead tired and already thinking about my afternoon nap.

2. I drink:
   a. Four to six glasses of water daily, and fresh organic vegetable and fruit juices weekly.
   b. Only the bottle of water I keep in the car.
   c. Only diet soda or iced tea.

3. I have a bowel movement at least once a day, usually within twenty-five to forty-five minutes of waking.
   a. Absolutely!
   b. Some days are better than others.
   c. I am often constipated.

4. I exercise regularly—three to five times a week for twenty-five to seventy-five minutes each time.
   a. Yes, it's an important part of my life.
   b. If I have the time I do.
   c. Never; I hate it.

5. My diet includes plenty of fresh (preferably organic) seasonal fruits and vegetables.
   a. Yes, I love eating healthy food and will go out of my way to do so.

b. I try to be conscientious, but I usually just grab whatever is around when I am hungry.

c. Does it count if it comes out of a can or is a week old?

6. I consider myself a moderate social drinker.

a. I drink fewer than seven alcoholic beverages a week (and not all in one night).

b. When I am in a social setting, it's easy to get carried away.

c. Who's counting, anyway?

7. I have a job that allows me to be my creative best, and I enjoy myself there.

a. Yes, I love my work.

b. I'm comfortable in my job, but I often fantasize about moving on.

c. I dread going to work every day.

8. I have a fun, supportive, stimulating social circle of friends who support me in being and doing my very best.

a. Yes, my friends are warm and supportive.

b. My friends are okay, but I am often left feeling dissatisfied.

c. No, my friends are difficult and often a source of stress.

9. My romantic and sexual needs are met, or at least I am getting closer to having them met by effective communication.

    a. Yes; although I do experience life's ups and downs, I feel happy.

    b. I have had my disappointments, and I feel discouraged most of the time.

    c. I don't even know what I want; I'm too busy to take the time to figure it out.

10. Outside work:

    a. I make time to pursue my hobbies.

    b. I seem to run a lot of errands and do a lot of chores but have no energy for anything else.

    c. I watch TV and surf the Web, mostly alone.

11. To me, inner reflection means:

    a. Making time to go within, meditate, and quiet my mind.

    b. Trying to stop my thoughts.

    c. Figuring out what I am going to have for dinner.

12. My body aches:

    a. Rarely; I am mostly free from nagging aches.

    b. When I awaken or at the end of the day.

    c. Always; it seems I always have a little ache somewhere.

13. On the whole, my life is:

    a. Happy and fulfilling.

    b. Generally okay; I'm not really sure how to make it better.

    c. In need of help.

14. I have a few extra pounds to lose:
   a. Not at all.
   b. On and off throughout my life.
   c. Don't ask, don't tell!

If you answered A to ten or more: You are a happy, ful-filled, balanced human being. Your healthy lifestyle is a priority for you, and it shows! You enjoy your work pursuits and understand the value of strong, evolving relationships with others. Acupuncture will help you maintain balance in your life. Your EnerQi is functioning at its highest frequency.

If you answered B to eight or more: You may feel like you ride shotgun through life. Although life is generally good and you don't have too many complaints, you know that you are capable of creating more for yourself. Becoming more balanced will put you back in the driver's seat, thus empowering you to be healthier and happier while raising your EnerQi vibration.

If you answered C to five or more: You feel more "off" than "on." You know it is time to make a change! You have nothing to lose and everything to gain. The sky is the limit for what you can create, if you take the time to explore who you are, what you want, and what you truly value. Begin your inner journey now! Change is truly the only constant in life, and once you have achieved balance, you will be open and welcome to change and growth.

Jing Essence and the
Ming Men Fire

In addition to having qi, we are also born with another very important power within us called *jing* essence. We inherit *jing* essence from our parents and their parents, and it determines our constitutional strength. Unlike qi, *jing* essence is much more difficult to strengthen, although it can be nourished through a healthy lifestyle. *Jing* essence is stored in the kidneys, whereas qi is stored throughout the body.

The kidneys also house the *ming men* fire, known as the Gate of Vitality. The most important job of the Gate of Vitality is to create heat and fire, which in turn creates the movement of energy and therefore gives us power (as with an engine). *Ming men* fire heats our body and allows the kidney essence to have the power to perform the daily tasks necessary for the body's proper functioning. The stronger the kidney qi, the better nourished and cared for the *jing* essence is.

For this reason, the kidneys are often referred to as the battery pack of the body. *Jing* essence is called upon as we go about our daily lives, sleeping, eating, and exercising. The big difference between qi and *jing* is that qi can be nourished and strengthened by a healthy lifestyle, but *jing* energy is more precious and cannot be re-created once it has expired. Death is the only available option because we are all born with a contained amount of *jing* essence. Once it is gone, so is life.

Think of *jing* essence as a deep well within us that our bodies' qi, blood, and oxygen draw from to fuel their inner strength and fire. Congenitally, some of us have stronger and deeper wells than others do; that is just the way biological inheritance works. Your natural *jing* essence is taken into consideration when qi is strengthened for a comprehensive approach to improving and sustaining your EnerQi.

Understanding the Meridians

Oriental medical practitioners believe that bodies are lined with vertical and horizontal, internal and external, invisible pulsating energy fields called *meridians*, which are thought to be electromagnetic. Our bodies' qi, blood, and oxygen charge the meridians. The qi travels along our meridians, internally and externally, forming channels for the movement and distribution of life force, up, down, in, and around the entire body. These meridians cover us, wrapping around the entire body and connecting to the blood, capillaries, muscles, tendons, joints, bones, internal organs, other meridians, genitals, limbs, brain, eyes, ears, nose, teeth, and mouth.

Energetically, twelve of these meridians are the body's main meridians, and two others are the body's master meridians. When our qi becomes blocked or stagnant, the result is an excess or a deficiency of qi, blood, or oxygen, which increases or decreases the activity of our bodily systems and affects our EnerQi. Our qi becomes blocked for a variety of reasons, including but not limited to poor nutrition, drug use, alcohol abuse, injury, lack of sleep, lack of movement, stress, mental outlook, excessive dampness, and cold or heat.

Stagnation: Blocked Qi

Stagnation and *blocked qi* are main buzzwords in Chinese medicine. The Chinese consider stagnation to be one of the body's "great evil entities." Evil entities in Chinese medicine are thought to be any environmental disease or physical malady in the body other than optimum health. Unfortunately, a lot of people suffer from stagnation.

There are five different kinds of stagnation: food, fluid, cold, qi, and blood. Any one of these can turn into heat and cause an inflammatory condition in the body.

Various shades of purple and various shades of blue on the body and/or the tongue indicate stagnation. These colors are not viewed as beneficial to overall health because they represent the reduced flow of blood, qi, and oxygen. They indicate to the practitioner that the body is not getting the nourishment and reinforcement it needs from within to support ongoing empowered healthy normal functioning.

Think of a pool of crystal-clear blue moving water. For the water in the pool to stay clean and free of harmful bacteria, it needs the movement from the current of the wind. This current circulates the water, keeps it clean, and keeps the energy moving freely. When the water is still with no movement, over time it becomes a dirty and smelly breeding ground for inflammation, illness, and bacteria—an "evil entity."

Herein lies the reason it is so important for us to give our bodies proper mental, spiritual, and physical care. When our qi becomes blocked, the movement that is necessary for circulation—which makes us strong and vibrant and keeps us healthy—is not available to nourish us properly to maintain good health.

The immune system and our general overall wellness are strong indicators of how balanced our qi is. How well is your immune system protecting you? Imbalanced qi can lead to pain, disease, and lethargy. Oriental doctors believe that the meridians are electromagnetic and that each one carries with it its own energetic qi vibration along these channels. The meridians serve as a grid for us to look for and distribute qi, blood, and oxygen within the organs, tendons, ligaments, nerves, and muscles, using pressure or puncture techniques. When the balance of the body's natural electromagnetic energy is restored through acupuncture, the body can heal itself and begin to function properly once again. (You'll learn more about acupuncture in the upcoming chapters).

Qi as a River

A useful analogy to help explain the concept of qi and the meridians through which it flows are to imagine that your body's internal workings are a network of streams, inlets, and estuaries of clean, clear water. Sticks, stones, leaves, or large rocks can get in the way of the flow of this water.

These obstructions are our physical and mental imbalances, life's travails—the bumps, bruises, hurts, and misunderstandings we all experience along the way. A weakened immune system, unchecked addictions, constant emotional upheaval, weight challenges, lack of exercise, restless or sleepless nights, and ongoing fatigue and lethargy can create a never-ending litany of weakness, aches, and pains. These symptoms are the body's way of telling us it has distress from the dis-ease we are experiencing within our bodies. It may be a matter of lifestyle choices, which proper diet, exercise, and sleep can remedy.

However, once obstructed, the water (or qi) is forced to take another pathway down the stream by going around the rocks or under the leaves. The water still makes its way down the stream, but not in the most effective or efficient manner. Often, not enough water is coursing through the stream, whereas at other times too much water causes flooding or pooling. Acupuncture needles placed by a skilled practitioner serve as a sweeping branch to brush the accumulated debris away and allow the water to continue in a smooth and timely flow.

In other words, acupuncture is the facilitation of the energetic transport of qi, blood, and oxygen throughout the body. The thin metal needles are used to facilitate balanced movement. This movement of energy is an ongoing function that happens all the time in all living humans and animals, but as you've just learned, this energetic exchange can become blocked. What makes acupuncture unique is the magnetic charge that the needles provide as they are inserted along the pathways. They form a strong electromagnetic current that shifts and changes, revitalizes, recharges, and energizes the body and its many functions. Complemented by acupuncture, other Oriental techniques help to strengthen the qi and restore balance to the body.

Getting Beyond "Not Sick"

My wife brought me to see Sheri for acupuncture. I wasn't really sick per se; I just did not feel great most days. My regular doctor did a complete workup and everything looked fine.

I'm a regular guy who works long hours as an attorney and gets together with the guys once a week to golf; I drink beer and have some red wine with dinner a few nights a week. I was about fifteen pounds overweight, and my wife began noticing that I was snoring louder than usual.

Sheri gave me a diet to follow that eliminated a lot of the sugar and unhealthy snacks I was eating. My new diet included morning green drinks, more vegetables, fresh fruits, and a lot less meat. I ate more fish, and one day a week I ate only beans, salad, vegetables, and seeds. (I felt like a bird at first.)

I came in for acupuncture every week for twelve weeks, and she had me commit to an exercise routine of at least four times per week with a trainer from my local gym. I also started taking an herbal powder twice a day that she made for me in her clinic. For a guy who wasn't sick, I was amazed at how much better I felt and continue to feel!

I have a lot more energy and am not nearly as tired at the end of the day. My back was always sore before, and I thought it was something I was going to have to just live with. I have had no back pain since the third time I had acupuncture. My snoring has improved, and I have lost twelve pounds. I feel like I did fifteen years ago when I was thirty-five.

I think I will give meditation a try next. I highly recommend this type of "lifestyle fix" for someone who needs a change.

—*J. M., fifty-year-old male*

Changing My Outlook

Four years ago, when I first tried acupuncture, I had a host of health issues. I was suffering from depression; I had a rash that covered my arms, legs, and torso; and I was experiencing irregular heartbeat, fatigue, and headaches. None of the physicians I had seen in the past seven years could tell me what I had or help me.

At my first meeting with Sheri, she suspected that one of my problems was a food allergy. She put me on a restricted diet, and within weeks I felt better. We also discovered that I have an autoimmune disease. With acupuncture treatments, my rash began to disappear, and my immune system is now much more stable. Acupuncture, herbs, and dietary and lifestyle modifications changed my outlook, and I now know I can live a long and healthy life. Words can never express my gratitude.

—*D. K., forty-seven-year-old female*

Opening Myself Up to Healing

I decided to try acupuncture because my shoulder had been bothering me for quite some time. None of the normal medicine was helping. Even an osteopath using nonmainstream techniques did not yield long-term results. I needed to try something else. Fortunately, I was in a period of self-discovery, working on personal and health issues for the first time in my life. I had lots of support at my church and had great friends, so I was ready to make new choices. Trying something new was part of loving myself and taking responsibility for my own health and well-being.

During my first acupuncture session, I was apprehensive because it was something I had never experienced before. When you open yourself up to healing—whether it's soul, spirit, physical, or emotional—one can feel very vulnerable. I found that my acupuncturist's manner and empathy, as well as her ability to connect with and relate to me while properly diagnosing the problem, were as important as the treatment itself.

By the end of the second session, I began to really see some effects from the treatment. I felt much more relaxed, I had more energy, and my overall outlook on life improved. Since that time, I have improved, and the original problem in my shoulder has been greatly alleviated.

—*B. L. S., male, late forties*

Chapter 2

Drawing from Nature: The Elements of EnerQi

Deep in their roots,
all flowers keep the light.

—Theodore Roethke

Oriental medicine draws from nature to diagnose internal medical challenges. We have all admired a great majestic tree. Your health is like that great majestic tree. The roots are your immune system, your qi essence, and the power of your qi essence. The branches of your tree are your subjective symptoms of a greater imbalance.

The problem is not in a bad branch; it actually lies in
the roots of the tree and within the soil that nourishes
the tree. What is the underlying cause of distress?
Let's take a look.

Root and Branch

I have a patient who suffered from terrible migraine
headaches (the branch). Rather than simply treat the headache, I looked at what else was going on within her ecosystem (i.e., her body) that could be the cause (the root) of
the headache. This patient is a very fit and physically active
forty-five-year-old female. Nevertheless, she experienced a
migraine every month, lasting a week at a time, for fifteen
years. She slept terribly and reported anxiety during the
same time frame. She also complained of poor digestion
and ongoing fatigue.

In considering the root and branch theory, I knew that
the headaches were a symptom and not the cause of the
dysfunction. Using acupuncture and herbs, I was able to
get her to sleep soundly for six to eight hours a night. That
alone decreased her anxiety level, and with my supervision
in collaboration with her doctor, she was slowly able to
wean herself off her antianxiety medication and sleeping
pills. I analyzed her nutrition and put her on a program

that included more warm vegetables, nourishing soups, and fewer cold salads.

Warmth activates the spleen which encourages and initiates better digestion and elimination. Once her sleep, anxiety, and digestion became more in balance, her hormones adjusted as well. Her ongoing fatigue started to improve once she was digesting better because she was able to get more nutrition from better food choices. The quality of her sleep was much more sound because she had less stomach distress, which had been contributing to keeping her awake and uncomfortable. She was able to incorporate daily walks into her life since she was less tired and had more energy. Without a doubt, exercise really helped her anxiety and stimulated the hormones that promote well-being. Voilà! Fewer headaches within one menstrual cycle!

I have been treating this patient for six months now, and she has experienced almost a complete cessation of migraines. More work is required for her body to become balanced, yet we have gotten halfway there by approaching treatment of the condition as a whole.

If you suffer from migraines or other ailments, you can expect lasting relief when your practitioner identifies and treats the *root cause* of your symptoms rather than the symptoms that branch from the root cause.

What's at the Root of the Chief Complaint?

I always listen very carefully to what my patients present as their chief complaint, while consistently exploring the deeper levels to uncover what is truly causing their imbalance. The "root and branch" diagnostic theory dictates from within you where we need to begin to balance and correct the disharmony. This means that your condition is not the cause of the dis-ease; it is merely the manifestation or branches of the true, underlying root cause (with the exception of a sports injury, sprain, or strain). If only symptoms are treated and the fundamental root cause is not addressed, it is like constantly bailing water out of a leaking boat rather than fixing the leak in the first place.

The elements of nature that Oriental medicine assigns to our pulses are the same ones used to explain the way our body functions. Think of your internal organs as a representation of the universe. We are taught that the heart is like the sun in the sky, the spleen is the soil covering the earth, the lungs are the sky or the atmosphere, the kidneys are the salty seas, and the liver is the circulating wind. The elements of fire, earth, metal, water, and wood symbolize the interrelationships of these organs.

We call this order of elements the *control and nourish cycle*. As you're reading about the elements and body functions below, keep in mind that the Eastern concepts of body functions and organ systems are different from the Western way of thinking. Acupuncturists take Western concepts into consideration but expand on them. For example, when I say *liver*, I'm speaking not only of the liver's functions of cleansing blood and digesting nutrients; in Oriental medicine, the liver's functions are more encompassing. An example of how the elements are used in diagnosis can be found in the concept of the twelve pulses and their relationship to one another. These relationships are interdependent, since each one feeds another.

To understand the control and nourish cycle, let's return to the analogy of the great strong tree planted in the earth. This tree gets much-needed energy to grow from clean oxygen in the air and thrives by the warmth of the sun and the quality of the soil. The soil feeds the roots so they can spread freely. The water from the rain and snow nourish and moisten these roots, which enable the trunk, bark, and branches to grow strong and flourish.

This cycle continues year after year, drawing upon and feeding upon these important elements in nature. Each of these elements depends on and helps others to nurture and grow. They are all connected to one another. This cooperation of elements allows for healthy qi and sustained longevity.

Fire, earth, metal, water, and wood exist in our material world. Each element carries within it its own yin and yang energy. The elements can function alone, but they work best when they act together because they depend on, assist, and act on one another. Because these elements need one another to function, if they are out of balance, one element can cause another to malfunction. We are only as strong as our weakest link.

These elements, like life itself, are in constant motion, cyclical and always changing. Oriental medicine assigns the elements to our internal organs, our outward extremities, and our psychological and emotional states. Each element, along with its associated organ, has a specific time of day or night for optimal functioning. This time factor serves as a check-and-balance system within the body. The elements help to paint an archetype of thought, word, and deed for the practicioner, who is using all the senses to make an accurate diagnosis. These archetypes are broad generalizations based on the characteristics of each element. Most people will have a true dominant element and one or two secondary elements that are active within the body at the same time.

Read the following descriptions of each of the elements; you may begin to see yourself, or someone close to you, functioning within these concepts. If you notice that you are experiencing any of the symptoms of the excess of an element, or you relate to feeling out of balance after reading about the elements you identify with, make a note of it. Then be sure to discuss your impressions with a qualified Oriental medical practitioner.

Fire Attributes

The organs of the fire element are the heart (yin), which is at its peak between 11:00 AM and 1:00 PM, and the small intestine (yang), which peaks between 1:00 and 3:00 PM. The fire element is known as the king because the heart pumps blood through the vessels to the entire body. The heart contains the spirit, also known as *shen*, which houses and controls the mind.

The small intestine plays a role in the body's water distribution process and metabolism. The small intestine separates the impure waste materials from the pure nutritious elements of foods. The pure elements are circulated throughout the body, and the impure elements are sent on to the large intestine, which is known as the receiver.

You are directly experiencing the heart element when you are feeling happy, laughing, or hearing the sound of laughter. The fire season is the early summer, the climate is hot, the direction is south, the color is red or pink, the taste is bitter, and the smell is scorched or burned. The tongue is the flower of the heart; this means that the tongue, especially the tip, can tell me the condition of a patient's heart element, and emotional state. For example, if you came for treatment with sores on your tongue, it would be a tip for your practitioner to pay attention to the heart element during treatment.

Fire personalities have an intimate, warm, open, expressive, and compassionate temperament. Their facial colors tend toward redness, whitish gray, or a pale, flushed face; their walk is bouncy and fast. The head or the chin will often be pointed, and they tend to have small hands. Their hair is usually curly or sparse. They can be active, energetic, smart, inventive, alert, and excitable, yet they are sometimes scattered. Fire types appreciate beauty, can have explosive tempers, and are prone to chaos (think of fireworks going off, with many colors filling the sky all at once).

Fire types are typically great talkers; crave hot, spicy foods (fire feeds fire); tend toward nervousness; and love fame and recognition. When there is an imbalance, they become excessively talkative, laugh inappropriately, and often miss social cues to stop and listen. This could be an indication of a *shen* disturbance.

An excess of the fire element also sometimes manifests as dizziness, a urinary tract infection, heart palpitation, or angina. Typically, there is sleep disturbance or dream-disturbed sleep. Uncontrollable laughter is often seen. Prolonged emotional sadness or mental illness is common. Excessive walking (i.e., walking for hours on end) strains the fire element.

Earth Attributes

The organs of the earth element are the spleen (yin), which is at its peak between 9:00 and 11:00 AM, and the stomach (yang), which peaks between 7:00 and 9:00 AM.

The spleen and the stomach are the main organs of digestion and assimilate food and fluids. These organs are collectively referred to as the center of the body.

The spleen regulates the blood and helps to keep it within its channels. It transforms food into nourishment and moves those nutrients upward to the stomach. The stomach regulates the sea of nourishment, performing the rottening and ripening process as it receives the food and moves nutrients downward. The earth element houses the thoughts and controls the flesh and the limbs. The mouth is the flower of the spleen and the stomach.

The earth's direction is the center, its climate is damp, and its smell is of sweetness and perfume. The emotion is pensiveness or deep thinking; the sound is of singing. You are directly experiencing the energy of the earth element when you taste sweetness; when you wear the colors yellow, orange, beige, or brown; or when you enjoy the days of late summer.

Earth types are relaxed, slow, sensitive, and sweet. They love pleasure and are generous, kind, calm, and extremely sensitive. Typically, but not always, the abdomen is chunky, large, and soft. The head and the jaw are often large and wide. Earth types have soft, cuddly flesh yet are full and muscular. The upper arm skin sometimes hangs below the muscle.

When they walk, earth types do not lift their feet very high (because they are grounded to the earth). They love to save, save, save, and they are often referred to as pack rats. They tend to love the simple things in life and are not exceedingly ambitious. They are deep thinkers who tend to chew their cud (i.e., they are mental ruminators). They always want more, especially of sugary treats.

You can tell when earth types are out of balance because they seem scattered, with confused thinking. They may have difficulty concentrating, often forgetting what they were doing or where they were going in the first place. A deficiency in the earth element weakens the spleen, causing dampness, indigestion, bloating, and tiredness after meals. In contrast, dryness weakens the stomach, which manifests as acid indigestion, ulcers, pain, or burning. Most deficient disorders in the body's center stem from the spleen; most excess disorders in the body's center stem from the stomach.

Excess sitting strains the earth element. When the spleen is weak, the body is unable to use the nutrients from food. This is often a result of a surplus of iced or cold foods and beverages or excessively spicy foods. This challenge can be corrected with a change of diet to include more appropriate food choices. Excessive worry injures and weakens the earth element.

Metal Attributes

The organs of the metal element are the lungs (yin), which peak between 3:00 and 5:00 AM, and the colon, or large intestine (yang), which peaks from 5:00 to 7:00 AM.

The metal element is known as the prime minister because it is in charge of the orderly rhythm of qi and breath in the body. The lungs are responsible for breathing and take in the qi from the air while governing the qi, or energy states, within the body. The lungs are the master of qi and govern the voice and the skin. The lungs house the corporeal soul, which is the physical part of the soul that manifests as feelings and sensations. The corporeal soul is linked to our breath and our ability to take long, deep, open, cleansing breaths.

The large intestine is called the minister of transportation and is responsible for elimination. It extracts water from the impure essence it receives from the small intestine, transports the liquid waste to the bladder, and excretes the solid leftover waste as stool. Those who are experiencing the energy of the metal element will often feel emotionally wistful. The metal sound is crying or whining; the season is autumn, and the climate is dry. The metal direction is west, the color is metallic or white, the taste is pungent or spicy, and the smell is fishy or rank. The nose is the flower of the lungs.

A metal temperament is often inspired, courteous, disciplined, refined, precise, formal, and happy after accomplishments. It is quite common for metal types to well up while watching a movie or hearing a sad story. This is a reflection of their sensitive souls. They typically have fine features with small bones, yet they have broad, strongly built bodies and square shoulders. They tend to walk slowly and deliberately and will sometimes have strong voices. Their health is reflected in the skin and the hair (which is shiny and bouncy), although they sometimes have a tendency toward dryness.

Metal types can be strict with themselves and others, are attached to their ideas, can be neurotic, and will not stop at a task until it has reached their idea of perfection, because they have strong wills. Too much talking weakens the metal element, as does excessive grief and melancholy.

A deficiency in the metal element often manifests as an inability to take deep, long breaths. Lung types are often uncomfortable with and have difficulty expressing feelings. The corporeal soul becomes weak because of an inability to take deep, cleansing breaths. Many metal types report tightness in the chest, asthma, and a compromised immune system. The lungs are the most delicate of the organs and are the first to be attacked by external pathogens (the common cold and the flu) when the body is weak. Rashes are common because the lungs control the metabolism within the body that distributes liquid to bathe and moisten the skin.

Water Attributes

The organs of the water element are the kidneys (yin), which are at their peak from 5:00 to 7:00 PM, and the bladder (yang), which peaks from 3:00 to 5:00 PM. The kidneys are responsible for reproduction, growth, and regeneration. They are said to be the ministers of health because of the importance of their role. The bladder is called the outlying district official; it controls and transports the body's fluids and excretes them.

Diagnosis always takes into consideration the health of the kidneys because they are the root of yin and yang in the body. The kidneys house our willpower. They also house the *ming men* fire, known as the Gate of Vitality, which is the source of the body's EnerQi and the power for all the internal organs. The most important job of the Gate of Vitality energy force is the creation of heat and fire, which causes the movement of energy and therefore creates power within us, like an engine. *Ming men* fire heats the body and allows the kidney essence to have the power to perform the daily tasks required for proper body functioning. For this reason, the kidneys are called the battery pack of the body, as was mentioned in Chapter 1.

You are experiencing the water element when you feel fear or hear the sounds of tiresome groaning and grumbling. The season is winter, the climate is cold, and the direction is north; the color is black, purple, or blue; the taste is salty, and the smell is rotten or putrid. The ears are the flower of the kidneys.

Water types are easygoing, calm, creative, ambitious, sensitive, sympathetic, and sometimes psychic. They are perceptive, aware, sharp in their thinking, loyal to their friends, eccentric, and are self-assured. They are flexible in their personalities. They can eat most things because they typically have strong digestive systems. Water types swing when walking and flow like waves. They can have round faces and bodies, with soft skin and thin, wiry frames. Typically, water types have difficulty holding on to body weight even though they are good eaters who are known as "grazers," always snacking throughout the day and the night.

Water types can be jumpy or easily startled, yet they love to lie around and lounge. They are prone to telling little white lies. The reflection of strong health within the water element can be found in the condition of the bones, marrow, brain, hair (premature graying and hair loss), teeth, inner ear, pupils, and lumbar region, which houses the kidney essence.

Overexposure to fright or fear weakens the water element. A deficiency in the water element can manifest as high- or low-frequency ear ringing, infertility, lower back pain, weak vision, confusion, apathy, and sorrow. If imbalanced, water types can run a very hot body temperature, with sweaty palms. They can become so hyper that they can't rest when they lie down, and they often have night sweats with restless sleeping. With a deficiency, they can also be clammy or chilly and will want to lie, shivering, in a curled fetal position to try to get warm. A kidney weakness will always show up as dark or gray circles under the eyes. With this weakness comes the need for a lot of rest, because water types tire easily from the time they are children. Children often fail to thrive and have higher incidences of asthma.

Any chronic condition will always involve the kidneys; your practitioner will seek to maintain the strength and vitality of the kidneys with every treatment. A lifestyle of excess will strain the water element. Exhaustion, excessive sexual activities, overexercise, long periods of standing, excessive drinking, and external attacks of cold (i.e., catching a chill) are common causes of long-term weakness. Women often have weak or no menstruation, and men often moan and groan in frustration about impotence, weak sex drive, or premature ejaculation. Both will have frequent occurrences of urination, especially at night. Chronic lower back pain is common.

Wood Attributes

The organs of the wood element are the liver (yin), which is at its peak between 1:00 and 3:00 AM, and the gallbladder (yang), which peaks from 11:00 PM to 1:00 AM. The liver is said to be the general within the body; its functions are to plan, organize, and coordinate among the organs. The liver stores the blood and regulates the movement and flow of qi within the body. It regulates the other organs because of its function of spreading qi. It houses the ethereal soul, which is said to influence our sense of direction in life, our emotions, and our capacity to plan life's pursuits. Another important function of the liver is to nourish and bathe the tendons, ligaments, muscles, and joints with moisture, allowing for suppleness and flexibility.

The gallbladder is named the judge because it is responsible for decision-making. The gallbladder stores and secretes bile, which is produced by the liver. It is said to purify yang energy, holding the pure and impure essence of the body.

You are experiencing the wood element when you feel anger or frustration, shout or hear shouting, and enjoy the season of spring. The wood climate is windy, the direction is east, the color is green or blue green, the taste is sour, and the smell is yeasty or musty. The eyes are the flower of the liver and, with the nails, reflect the health of the liver.

Wood personalities are regal in nature, hardworking, talkative, confident, competitive, precise, and bold achievers. A lot of wood element body types are thin, wiry, and compact, with firm and tight muscles, or they can be quite muscular and strong, with broad shoulders. In excess, wood types are easily irritated and prone to anger, moodiness, and temperamental behaviors, such as temper tantrums and yelling.

Wood types are known to have an exaggerated sense of self-importance. This behavior is referred to as being "liverish" and is very easy to spot. They are the bores in restaurants that yell at the staff for forgetting their water. They are the parents who become easily frustrated, are undeniably aggravated, lose patience, and scream loudly at their children for the slightest transgression. They have a tendency to worry, find it hard to relax, and can be prone to depression.

Meditation, long walks, running, yoga, having lots of fun, and staying up into the wee hours of the morning relax and make wood types happy. Most wood-element people characterize themselves as "night owls," although they really need to be in bed by 11:00 PM. Otherwise, they get an energetic second wind and will happily be up until 2:00 AM because the liver is regenerating during this time.

Those with wood disharmony are always attracted to and love the color purple (the color of royalty). They wear it often (even to the clinic for treatments) and are known to even paint their homes in various shades of purple. Depression and anger disturb the quality of wood's functioning, which is otherwise free flowing. (The Chinese character for the liver signifies flowing and free). Many women suffer from liver qi disharmony (stagnation) because its function is so closely related to the storage of blood; hence its connection to premenstrual syndrome.

Excessive reading strains the liver; walking is the exercise of the liver. When there is a weakness in the gallbladder, the person will often be indecisive and timid. Deficient wood types have trouble deciding what to wear, what to eat, what to do, where to go, or even whether they should bother to go at all.

When the wood element is imbalanced, it is common to see neck and shoulder tension, headaches, high blood pressure, gas, stomach cramps, or a very tight stomach with nausea (before, during, and after eating). A sensation like a pit in the throat is often felt (this is called plum-pit qi). Urinary tract infections and prostatitis are common. Yellowish eyes, uncontrolled shaking, and restless leg syndrome are sometimes present. With a wood imbalance, it is not uncommon for patients to be diagnosed with Bell's palsy and other neuralgias. Patients often have vertical ridges in their fingernails.

As you can see, there is a very strong and vital yin-yang relationship among the organs. One cannot function without the help of the other. The temperatures within the elements vary, based on excess or deficiency, manifesting their balance or imbalance according to the element's climate. Temperatures are important to take into consideration when your practitioner is diagnosing and treating.

Referring to the cycle of life, the ancient texts say that fire renews the earth and is extinguished by water, earth creates metal and is penetrated by wood, metal holds water and is melted by fire, water nurtures wood and is contained by earth, and wood feeds fire and is cut by metal.

You will be able to identify a small part of yourself in each of the elemental characterizations. A good practitioner will be able to ascertain which parts of these characterizations make up the most of who you are and work from there to create balance and harmony.

Gaining a Higher Level of Health and Well-Being

At age thirty-six, shortly after my first and only pregnancy, I developed exercise-induced asthma that quickly worsened. It seemed that everything and nothing exacerbated my symptoms. Worse yet, the medications I was prescribed caused miserable side effects. While taking inhaled steroids and an allergy medication, I experienced cloudy thinking, blurred vision, disturbed sleep patterns, and anxiety. The treatment was as bad as the disease, which continued to worsen.

I had never known anyone who received acupuncture other than an acquaintance who received treatment for hormonal problems. Out of desperation I decided to try acupuncture, although this was a very different path from the one I followed as an educated professional with a bachelor's of science in nursing and a law degree. I was not so much skeptical as I was uninformed.

Within three months, I had stopped taking the inhaled steroids and the allergy medication. Within one year, I noticed that I was back to using my inhaled steroids only before exercise and not with every change in the weather and every single viral illness. Furthermore, I was overjoyed at the unintended—for me—benefits of acupuncture. My atypical, atopic dermatitis, present for more than ten years, had lessened in severity. The mood swings and many other physical symptoms I experienced as a result of early menopause were muted. I was sleeping more deeply and restfully even though I had been a lifelong insomniac.

There are many illnesses, syndromes, and conditions that I now know, as a result of personal experience as well as reading and research, are helped by acupuncture. It is a real therapy that made a real difference in my life, and it has helped me to gain a higher level of health and well-being."

—*R. H., female, mid-forties*

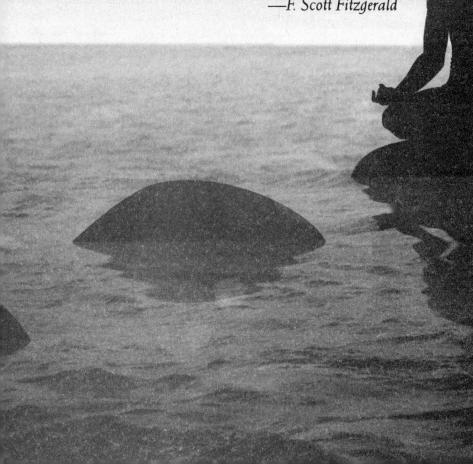

PART II

Align

THE WORLD ONLY EXISTS IN YOUR EYES—
YOUR CONCEPTION OF IT. YOU CAN MAKE IT
AS BIG OR AS SMALL AS YOU WANT TO.

—*F. Scott Fitzgerald*

Chapter 3

Restoring Balance with Diet, Herbs, and Homeopathics

There is but one temple in the universe,
and that is the body of man.

—Novalis

Just as people have qi circulating through their bodies, food also has its own qi vibration. Food is medicine. It restores and enlivens us. When we eat, we are consuming the qi of the food. It is very important to eat fresh fruits and vegetables because they are alive with vitality and contain large amounts of phytonutrients.

Their EnerQi complements and strengthens our own. Phytonutrient foods carry with them vibrant, powerful energy from the yin of the earth, the yang of the sun, and the oxygen in the atmosphere.

A diet of white flour and refined sugars does not have enough nourishment to keep you vital and glowing with powerful EnerQi, because refined foods lack blood and qi-producing nutrients. Bagels alone do not a meal make!

It is important to find the nutritional plan that works best for your body's needs. Nutritional wellness must be addressed by first looking at your diet. If you eat a variety of healthy whole foods and organic, chemical-free fresh fruits and vegetables in the colors of the season, you will be healthier in the long run and get most of your nutritional needs met. Supplements are best taken in moderation. If you are taking more than two or three a day, seek out a health professional to advise you.

Herbs are a natural medicine and should be treated as such. They are potent and powerful. Herbs can interact in a positive or negative way with any prescriptions, foods, or other supplements you are taking. Make sure you are working with an educated herbalist before embarking on any herbal remedy plan. The same advice is true for homeopathic medicines, which are based on the many plants, flowers, and essences in nature. They too can interact with any supplement, food, or herbal medicine you are taking. Seek professional advice when self-diagnosing or before embarking on any new natural health regimen.

The Keys to a Healthy Diet

The key factors in a healthy diet are not only *what* you eat but also how often and how much.

How Often to Eat

Ideally, it is best to eat every three hours throughout the day to keep your EnerQi and metabolism actively burning; eating often is like adding fuel to a burning fire. This method of eating can be thought of as the nondiet. This is a healthy and sensible way to enjoy a variety of food choices—eating small amounts of delicious foods to maintain a fit, healthy physique.

So rather than eating gargantuan meals, become a healthy "grazer." By eating every three hours, you will notice that your energy, thought processes, and emotions are more balanced throughout the day. People often counterintuitively think that by not eating they will lose weight; however, not eating causes your metabolism to slow down to a crawl because it conserves calories to use as EnerQi, or fuel. By eating regularly, you will add enough fuel to power your body, and it will release fat stores. You will find that you will begin losing the extra weight you have been carrying around.

Food takes on a different meaning as you naturally slow down and enjoy the tastes and the textures of what you are eating. You will also find that you are able to stop eating when you are satiated and before you are stuffed. Your next meal is coming right up when you are eating every three hours.

About Portion Sizes

An ideal meal portion is approximately the size of your palm. How much you eat, ideally, is in direct relation to the number of calories you need to maintain an active lifestyle and a healthy weight for your bone structure and height. If you have further questions about portion size, make an appointment to see a professional nutritionist or a practitioner who also specializes in nutrition who can work with you to determine an ongoing nutritional plan.

A small serving of protein, high-fiber foods (legumes, or beans), and a variety of fresh steamed seasonal vegetables, fresh fruits, nuts, or a garden salad make up most meals in a healthy eating plan.

A healthy snack might be one of the following:

- 6–8 almonds, Brazil nuts or cashews
- Half a cup of yogurt
- 2 ounces of hummus with whole-grain carb
- 1 rice cake

- 1 glass of fresh vegetable juice
- 1 small piece of fruit
- Almond butter on apple slices
- A few stalks of celery
- A palm-sized portion of fresh fruit with nuts
- A few dried fruit slices
- 2 ounces of string cheese, cottage cheese, or yogurt
- A coconut smoothie with kale and spinach
- Sliced turkey, chicken, or fish
- Avocado
- Beans
- Fresh salad greens
- Broth-based soup

These are all good foods that will fuel your body for activity throughout the day.

The key to success is to be organized when you shop and to have what you need on hand in your home or at your workplace when you are hungry.

Moderation and Variety

Another key to a healthy diet is moderation and variety. There is no one-size-fits-all approach to diet because we are each unique. As you learn to listen to your body, you will find that you eat when you are hungry, consume moderate portions, and crave the foods that your body needs.

Adding variety and eating moderately are good ways to get out of a food rut. Be open to trying new nutrient-rich foods and enjoying a variety of your nutrient-rich favorites. A balance of protein, carbohydrates, and fats is essential for good nutrition. A vegetarian diet is acceptable as long as the proper amounts of vegetable protein, fats, and carbohydrates are in balance.

Research and incorporate superfoods in your diet. Superfoods are just what they sound like: foods that have an abundance of disease-fighting nutrients and antiaging and immune-building properties. I have included some in the food lists below.

The following are seven heart-healthy high-protein foods:

- 1 cup of steamed soybeans or edamame
- 1 cup of cooked regular, whole-wheat, or wheat-free pasta
- 1 cup of cooked kidney beans
- 1 large egg
- 1 ounce of almonds, cashews, walnuts, Brazil nuts, or pumpkin seeds
- 1 medium slice of tofu
- 1 cup of cooked spinach, kale, Swiss chard, or other leafy greens

When you pair a little bit of protein with your carbohydrates, you will feel fuller longer. Don't be afraid to add a little bit of "good" (unsaturated) fat to your diet. Fat in your diet does not equate to fat on your body. A variety of the right kinds of fat—unsaturated omega-3 fats such as coconut oil, avocado, flaxseed, nut oils, and olive oil—are essential brain foods that nourish the skin and the hair and are vital anti-inflammatory and antiaging agents. Include antiaging herbs as well as seasonal organic fruits and vegetables in your meal preparation. There are many choices to pick from; here a few powerful choices to consider:

- Eggplant
- Red and green bell peppers
- Basil
- Brussels sprouts
- Tomatoes
- Blackberries
- Potatoes
- Avocado
- Broccoli
- Cabbage
- Carrots
- Kale
- Sweet potatoes

If you have arthritis, however, you may wish to avoid the vegetables in the nightshade family (i.e., eggplant, bell peppers, tomatoes, and potatoes), which can cause inflammation in your tendons and joints.

Fuel your body throughout the day by starting with breakfast. Your first meal of the day does not have to be large, just nutritious. Oatmeal is an excellent choice because studies show that oats lower "bad" cholesterol (LDL) and slow the rise of blood glucose after eating. Eating oatmeal lowers your blood pressure, and the fiber leaves you feeling fuller for longer.

Other breakfast choices that are delicious and light before a morning workout, as well as a great way to start the day, are the following:

- A morning smoothie made without sugar and served at room temperature or cool, but not cold. Some recommended ingredients are coconut milk, almond or cashew milk, or soymilk; kale or spinach; fresh berries or seasonal fruit; Greek yogurt, chlorella powder or whey powder; and chia seeds.

- Whole-grain toast or wheat-free toast with peanut butter or almond butter

- Eggs

- Warm miso soup with brown rice

- Kale and brown beans

- A handful of Brazil nuts or almonds mixed into some Greek yogurt

Once you open up to eating moderately and consuming a variety of foods that are good for you, you'll really start enjoying your new way of eating.

Dining out can be quite easy when you know how to order and make special requests, if necessary. Most restaurants offer a vegetable of the day, fresh salads, and a protein source—all of which you can order without the sauce or the dressing. Consider asking for fresh lemon, vinegar, and olive oil, instead of dressing, which often contains sugar or chemicals.

It is important to think of these changes to your diet as a permanent and positive lifestyle choice and not just another fad diet that is doomed to failure. This is a plan you can live with and love forever. Think of this as the "slow-the-aging-process inner-power plan"!

No one can be perfect, so when you do feel the need to splurge, enjoy it. Just start over as soon as possible on your healthy food path. With this attitude, you will begin to feel much more in balance, and your EnerQi vibration will reflect this positive change to eating well.

Clean, Seasonal Eating

It's always a good idea to eat fresh, in-season, preservative-free, organic foods. In the summer, choose a light cooling meal of fresh seasonal fruits or salads daily; in the winter, choose warm nourishing qi-enhancing foods such as steamed vegetables, including root vegetables; all varieties of squashes, soups, and stews; and hot vegetable casseroles with or without meat. These are all nourishing foods available in the winter. Be sure to wash all vegetables and fruits very well.

As you become more accustomed to eating fresh fruits and vegetables, you will notice that every season has its own offering; eat those seasonal offerings whenever possible. By eating whole healthy foods, you supply clean, clear EnerQi and sustenance to your body's vibrating root system.

The following is one of my favorite nourishing soups. Enjoy it piping hot in the winter or serve it cool in the summer, using a variety of seasonal colorful vegetables in the preparation.

Seasonal Cleansing Soup

· ·

1 gallon filtered or purified water

3 cups (or more) chopped seasonal vegetables, including
 dark leafy greens and/or tomatoes

1 cup chopped leeks, scallions or onions
 (more or less to taste)

1 garlic clove, chopped (more or less to taste)

1 large handful chopped fresh parsley and, or cilantro

Juice of 1 lemon or lime

Sea salt and pepper (to taste)

① Bring water to a boil in a large stockpot. Add chopped
vegetables, scallions, leeks or onions, and garlic and
allow to simmer for 15 minutes.

② Remove from heat and allow the vegetables to blanch
until the water cools. Add parsley and, or cilantro and
lemon or lime juice. Season with sea salt and pepper.

③ Reheat before serving. Sip warm, at room temperature,
if desired, or drink chilled in the summer.

④ Throughout the week, add to the stockpot or your
individual bowl any of the following: fish, chicken, saf-
fron rice, quinoa, lentils, or a poached egg. Feel free
to experiment with any garden herbs. As long as your
choices are healthy, you can't go wrong.

Expanding Waistlines

We learn from newspapers, magazines, news reports, and our own communities that obesity is a huge problem. We are finding more and more overweight children and adults than ever before in our society. We are slowly realizing the problem and looking for change; we understand that we can no longer ignore our own growing waistlines or those of our children or our parents. This expansion puts us at risk for pain, disease, needless shame, and discomfort. Fortunately, when it comes to diet, knowledge is the kind of power that can save a life.

When I see an overweight, lethargic person, I see a malnourished person who eats the wrong types of foods, in the wrong amounts, at the wrong times, in the wrong combinations. I always make an effort to spark a renewed interest in mindful, healthy eating in my patients, and I assure you that you can create delicious, interesting, healthy meal choices and, as a result, feel empowered, become healthier, and be in a better position to achieve your best. Remember, food is your fuel. Your body is a vibrant system that is nourished by your food choices. Share this knowledge with those you love and care for.

The EnerQi Eating Plan

The following is the EnerQi nutritional eating plan that I recommend on a regular basis to my patients for balancing their qi and raising their EnerQi vibration. My patients often tell me how great they feel after implementing these ideas into their food lifestyle.

Eat fruits, herbs, vegetables, beans, and grains according to the seasons. Nature supplies us with the proper nutrients we need in her choice of colors. Have you ever noticed how the colors of the vegetables change from summer to winter? These colors reflect the phytochemical content of the food. Phytochemicals are intelligent micronutrients that absorb the sun's energy. They are anticarcinogenic, anti-inflammatory, immune boosting, and mood modulating.

In the summer heat, you'll find cooling white corn and light green cucumbers that can be eaten raw or cold. In the winter chill, you'll find nourishing orange pumpkins and squashes that must be cooked and are usually eaten warm or hot. Seasonal eating is using the concept of interdependent energies to balance yin and yang at their best.

The following are some basic rules for healthy eating:

- Rotate what you eat; choose something different today from what you ate yesterday or the day before.

- Always strive to eat a balanced diet; this includes a healthy portion of protein, carbohydrates, and fats. If you are a vegetarian, you can add protein to your diet through tofu, tempeh, legumes, and nuts. (Beans and rice together equal 99 percent pure protein.)

- Reduce your intake of fatty fried foods, sugar, and alcohol.

- Focus on nutrition rather than on calories.

- Get as many nutrients from your food choices as you can; supplements are best used in addition to, not instead of, a healthy diet.

- Rotate your supplements and herbal preparations. It is never a good idea to stay on the same formulation for an extended period, unless prescribed by a healthcare practitioner. With supplements, less is definitely more.

- Make sure you include high-fiber foods (legumes, seeds, nuts, oats, and bran) as well as seasonal fruits and vegetables in your diet. This will increase your elimination rate, which allows toxins to pass through your body and reduces your cholesterol levels. A good daily dose of fiber is 25 grams for women, 35 grams for men. You might need to build up your fiber rate slowly yet steadily as your body learns to digest these additions to your diet. Chia seeds are a great way to get more fiber in your diet.

- Choose a high-calcium diet, which studies show reduces fat absorption in the body and contributes to weight loss. Green leafy vegetables, yogurt, and low-fat hard cheese are high in calcium; the recommended daily dose of calcium is 1,200 milligrams paired with 600 milligrams of magnesium, and this is ideally gotten through food.

- Monitor your salt intake.

- Monitor your saturated fat intake and avoid trans fats completely.

- Don't be afraid of healthy fat. Fresh nuts and nut butters can add important nutrients to your body. Healthy fat plays a role in reducing heart disease and balancing the nervous system. Experiment with the variety of sources of healthy unsaturated fat available on the market. Coconut oil, for instance, is rich in omega-6 oil, which fights free-radical damage in the body and benefits the skin by slowing down the effects of aging.

- Reduce your level of cortisol (the stress hormone) through the intake of omega-3 fatty acids; choose walnut and ground flaxseed in addition to liquid or encapsulated cod liver oil. Chia seeds and fish are also good sources of omega-3. This will improve your body's production of DHEA (dehydroepiandrosterone), which will enhance your memory and reduce inflammation. A benefit is enhanced moisture in the skin and hair.

- Make sure you get enough vitamin D, which boosts immunity, protects the body from cancer and osteoporosis, and safeguards the heart. Fifteen minutes of

sunshine daily on exposed skin can provide enough
of a dose; including mushrooms in your diet can be
helpful, since they synthesize vitamin D; or you can
take 1,000 IU daily in supplement form if you cannot
get adequate sun exposure. The benefits are improved
sleep, shining vitality, and enhanced immunity.

- Eat tomatoes to get lycopene, which has been shown
to protect the skin from the sun's harmful rays by
attaching to key cells on the skin's surface. Lycopene
synthesizes with vitamin D through sunshine, allowing a deeper penetration of protection into your skin
and replenishing your skin's elasticity.

- Take vitamin B12, which is essential for stress
reduction and which also supports the immune
system. The sublingual (under the tongue) form is
most easily assimilated. You can safely take 1,000
micrograms a day for up to two months; then it
is advisable to take a break.

- Get enough antioxidants in your diet. Vitamin E,
vitamin C, and selenium are the main power play-
ers. They attack damaging free radicals; recharge the
cells; protect proteins, fats, carbohydrates, and DNA;
and assist in the formation of antioxidant enzymes,
which protect blood cells from oxidative damage.

- Include sunflower seeds, almonds, hazelnuts, wheat
germ, and safflower oil in your diet for more vitamin E.

- Fortify your vitamin C stores with citrus, kiwi, straw-berries, peppers, and tomatoes.

- Boost your selenium intake with whole grains, nuts, seafood, and lean meats.

- Get a daily dose of zinc, especially if you are male; it is a very important mineral for the prostate. Good sources are a large handful of unsalted pumpkin seeds, whole grains, red meat, poultry, baked beans, chickpeas, cashews, and almonds.

The above recommendations will help you begin your nutritional lifestyle; however, it is always best to schedule a complete consultation with your family practitioner to make sure your particular nutritional needs are reviewed and a customized plan is created.

A Rainbow of Fruits and Vegetables

A British study confirmed that the more fruits and vege-tables we eat daily, the happier, more energized, and calmer we will feel.

Buying healthy, organic produce has never been easier or more fun. Many of the local farmer's markets, which are usually held on the weekends in the warmer months, carry organic produce from local farms. They also have live music, family play areas, picnic tables, and other goods to purchase. If outdoor markets are unavailable to you, visit your local grocery or natural foods store.

A variety of vegetables, vegetable juices, fruit juices, and smoothies are a wonderful way to vitalize our cells and give our bodies the extra boost of oxygenation that serves as rocket fuel for the blood cells. If you don't have a juicer or a blender, there are several fantastic organic green powders on the market that can be stirred into fresh water, or you can use store-purchased fresh juices.

Fresh daily seasonal vegetables, fermented foods such as sauerkraut, umeboshi plums, and daikon radish in vinegar help to alkaline the body's delicate pH balance, reducing an acidic state. Disease loves to linger in an acidic environment within the body, which also often causes anxiety and sleepless nights.

The more fresh organic fruits and vegetables we eat, the less we will crave processed foods and sugar. Organic is always the best choice since there are many pesticides and chemical sprays used during the nonorganic growing process that can cause disturbing side effects.

Take the time to gently scrub fruits and vegetables before consuming them. Add a teaspoon of apple cider vinegar to four cups of water and let the vegetables soak before using them to help remove any residue.

When steaming or sautéing vegetables, do so lightly at a lower heat, because using less heat preserves the nutrients. It's a good idea to keep your fruit and vegetables clean and ready in the refrigerator. This way, when you are hungry and ready for a quick snack, they will be the first food item you reach for.

Use vegetables and fruits as delicious dipping snacks paired with hummus, yogurt, cottage cheese, olive oil, peanut or almond butter, pesto sauce, beans, cheese slices, or olives.

Everything we put into our bodies has an effect on what we have going on outside our bodies. Give it a try. Make every meal a rainbow of fresh fruits and vegetables. Substitute empty calories for calories that count. Remember, your body is a vibrant energetic power source, your own beautiful temple.

How Herbs and Homeopathics Complement a Healthy Diet and Lifestyle

Herbs are incredibly powerful natural plant medicines of the earth. The same is true for homeopathics and the Bach flower remedies (dilutions of flower material developed by homeopath Edward Bach in the 1930s). These remedies beneficially affect our mental, physical, and spiritual selves. There are many wonderful over-the-counter formulations that you can take that will enhance the lives of you and your family. Choices include capsules, sublingual drops, lactose pellets, tonic teas, tonic foods, and healing salves or lotions.

Herbal and homeopathic medicines are to be chosen carefully and used only in addition to acupuncture and a healthy lifestyle, not in lieu of them. Many profound miracles may occur with the use of herbal and homeopathic medicines. Mistakes can be made when they are not used properly. Without proper guidance, people can misdiagnose themselves and, as a result, use the wrong herbal or homeopathic medicine and/or a faulty preparation and become ill.

Many well-known pharmaceuticals are made of herbal compounds. It is *very important* to study and research carefully the nature, taste, and indication of the herb or homeopathic remedy you are considering taking if you are self-diagnosing and self-medicating. Make sure you know the contraindications of each herb or homeopathic remedy you are considering—that is, how it may interact with supplements or pharmaceuticals that you are currently taking and with the foods that you are eating.

Remember that what is best for you might not work similarly for your family members or your pets. Check with a practitioner before embarking upon a complex herbal or homeopathic protocol.

It is never a pretty sight when a patient shows up in my clinic carting a huge shopping bag filled with myriad products that he or she has been taking. These products, while very beneficial taken separately or in moderation, can often cause harm or discomfort when they are mixed with other herbal or nutritional supplements or taken in too large a dose. Avoid this mistake. Use care and caution when taking herbal or homeopathic remedies.

An education in acupuncture includes training in the formulation of Chinese herbal medicines. Herbs are prescribed based on individual needs and conditions. Herbal medicine is not for everyone or for the treatment of every disease. Talk with your practitioner if you are interested in embarking on an herbal program to see whether it is a good fit for you.

Getting My Life Back

I was a 340-pound overweight man with diabetes, high blood pressure, breathing problems, and sleep apnea. I was also very depressed. I had never tried acupuncture and was very skeptical. I was at a point, though, that something had to change, and I knew I needed help or I was going to die.

Through changes in my diet and lifestyle, along with weekly acupuncture and counseling sessions, I am proud to say that I have successfully lost 140 pounds. A new person has emerged from my old self! It has been a lot of hard work but an incredible journey. The acupuncture has helped me with my anxiety issues. I have been able to regain my energy and lower my blood pressure, and I can once again breathe without difficulty. My metabolism is able to work efficiently, and while I still have some work ahead of me, I couldn't have done it without my regular acupuncture treatments and the wisdom that Oriental medicine offers.

—*B. I., male, late forties*

Enjoying Rest and Rejuvenation

I have severe osteoarthritis in my left hip and moderate to severe osteoarthritis in my right hip, plus a bone spur in my left heel. My qualitative impression of acupuncture is that it seems to have arrested the deterioration at a minimum. I seem to walk with less of a limp than formerly. An unexpected side benefit is that I have also been able to lose thirty pounds that I was not able to shed previously.

I have been receiving acupuncture treatments and nutritional counseling for more than six months. The acupuncture sessions provide me with almost a trancelike-quality period of rest and rejuvenation, a feeling of overall well-being. The results have been wonderful in the context of my overall hectic personal and professional lifestyle. The respite is something that I look forward to every week, and the feeling of relaxation and well-being that it generates lasts throughout the day but also helps create a sense of greater calmness throughout the week. I benefit from my acupuncture treatments and always look forward to my visits and naps.

—*M. R., male, late sixties*

Chapter 4

Magnifying EnerQi with Exercise

When one must, one can.

—Yiddish proverb

One of the biggest challenges I notice in my practice is that many patients are suffering from a lack of *intentional* exercise. Walking from the car in the parking lot into the restaurant is just not enough! I joke with my patients that lifting the fork from the plate to the mouth is not a good workout. I tell them that we need at least twenty-five to sixty minutes of exercise five times a week, depending on age and overall health.

Exercise supports detoxification in the body and stimulates blood circulation, lymphatic flow, respiration, and sweat. Sweating releases toxins from our bodies. Exercise helps our internal organs to function properly, because it regulates our digestion and elimination and stimulates the kidneys to release unwanted chemicals from the waste within.

Think about exercise the way you think about your job. Most of us get up five days a week and go to work. It's just what we do. For the most part, we don't make excuses about being too busy, too tired, or not in the mood. Even if that's true, we still go to work. We show up because we have to.

If you think about exercise the same way you think about going to work, it becomes nonnegotiable. It's your *job* to keep your body healthy and fit. Most people who participate in regular exercise feel better physically, sexually, emotionally, mentally, and spiritually. Exercise stimulates endorphins in the brain, which makes us feel energized calm, happy and relaxed. Regular exercise empowers and magnifies our vitality. Rather than making us feel tired, the right kind of regular exercise enlivens the body and increases hormone production.

Make sure you drink enough water before, during, and after your exercise. Water enhances the carrying of unwanted toxins from the cells, blood, and lymph system through sweating and elimination.

Great Ways to Get Exercise

Walking outside while breathing deeply is an excellent way to get exercise. If winter conditions keep you inside, think about joining a gym or getting together with a friend to dance or enjoy some other form of movement. Using DVDs and online videos is a great way to ensure a fun and interesting exercise routine.

There are so many options: free weights, exercise bands, core-strength-building exercises, Pilates, jump rope, Zumba, Nia, dance classes, barre work, cycling indoors and out, elliptical machines, supervised obstacle courses, martial arts, tai chi, *qigong* (pronounced "chee-gung"), yoga, outdoor hiking, and rock-climbing walls. These are just a few of the many fun and empowering ways in which you can get out in the world, be creative in your exercise program choices, have fun, and explore your body's capabilities for feeling healthy, alive, and enlivened. With a little experimentation, you can easily find a class or a method of exercise that is right for you.

Qi, blood, and oxygen cannot move freely to nourish our bodies if there is a lack of movement, prolonged stiffness, or stagnation within the body. So stretching is another must. Flexibility is a very important component of fitness; it is vital that our tendons, ligaments, and important connective tissue remain supple as we age. It is paramount to the health and ease of movement within our bodies. With every stretch, you move your qi, blood, and oxygen, which nourishes your mind; supports the tissues, ligaments, and skeletal system; and leaves you feeling energized, refreshed, and ready to meet your day.

To increase the vitalization of your body's qi, blood, and oxygen, make time to dry-brush your body once a week before a bath or shower. Use a natural loofah or a dry brush; starting from your heels, rub up toward your heart in small circular motions, and cover your entire body from bottom to top.

After a workout, try a warm-water Epsom salt bath. Soaking is a great way to relax the muscles. Steambaths and saunas are another way to relax and detox. Make sure you drink enough water before and after so you do not get dehydrated.

Schedule a regular massage when you know that you will be able to let yourself relax. Start with gentle pressure, and make sure the soles of your feet and the palms of your hands are included. As you get used to the sensations, you can request deeper pressure over time.

Make a Commitment

Make a commitment to get moving. You must stretch yourself figuratively and metaphorically in order to expand your life. Somehow, some way, do something that lengthens and moves your body. Anything that will elevate your heart rate (within your own margin of safety), promote sweat, and cause your face to become lightly flushed will do the trick. It also helps to remember to maintain a pleasant expression throughout the experience.

Have fun with your choice. You have to be willing and ready to incorporate exercise into your life. That's when it will become tolerable—something you look forward to and have a good time doing, a gift you give to yourself. When energy moves, change becomes apparent in your body and in your life almost immediately.

Your Body as a Garden

After the long cold winter, when the garden has been left untended, the soil is hard, weeds pop up everywhere, and the new green growth cannot be seen, even though it is there but just obscured. When one begins to work the soil a bit, breaking it up, pulling weeds, watering and fertilizing, the new sprouts begin to shoot up out of the ground. If you haven't tended your "garden" in a while, it is never too late to start. Begin your maintenance process now. Nurture your body as you would your garden and give it the care it needs to be strong and healthy for you.

Sexual health is also of great importance in moving and maintaining healthy qi. Make the most of your experience—orgasms move energy and enhance your EnerQi. If you don't use your natural sexual functions, your ability to do so can become compromised. (Sexuality is discussed more in Chapter 7, in the context of relationships.)

Oriental Forms of Exercise

In China, in the early morning hours, people from all walks of life are out in the parks doing tai chi and *qigong*. These exercises are designed to keep the body strong and supple, provide relaxation, and allow the mind to stay clear throughout the aging process. My master, Dr. Tan, practices regularly and teaches all his students and many of his patients qi-building techniques that strengthen the mind and the body.

Yoga is another great way to enhance your flexibility and relax your mind. Tai chi, *qigong*, and yoga all allow us to work at an individual pace and achieve our personal best through the practice. There is no competition or race to finish. Our bodies, like life itself, are in an ongoing, changing, evolving process. Make sure you are enjoying your journey.

Incorporating Exercise

I never thought about exercise as something I could really enjoy.

Sheri strongly suggested that I find an activity that interested me and do it up to five times a week.

At first I honestly did not know if I could commit to a regular program and make it a priority. The funny thing is that after four weeks, I really felt better. I was happier and had more energy. I look better in and out of my clothes after just three months. My sexual desire is a lot stronger, and my digestion is working so much better.

When the weather is nice, I spend time walking or jogging outdoors. I purchased a stationary bike for my den. I can watch the news while I am riding toward health.

I definitely do feel better, and I now see myself making a lifetime commitment.

—M. C., *fifty-five-year-old male*

Chapter 5

Using Your Mind to Fine-Tune Your Vibration

He who cannot change the
very fabric of his thought will never
be able to change reality
and will never, therefore,
make any progress.

—Anwar Sadat

In Oriental medicine, we have a saying that applies powerfully to us all: The mind leads the qi. In other words, your mind acts as the master, and your qi is the servant. By reframing your thoughts and emotions, keeping your attitudes positive, and making your behaviors empowered, you will tune your inner energetic essence to a higher level. As you fine-tune your body's EnerQi vibration, you will notice that you attract positive changes in your life and your health.

Think of your body as a pathway, a stream that carries your own channel of energy fields. Your thoughts start the chain of command, the beginning of your qi stream. Qi begins in your mind and takes directions from your thoughts, which instruct it to flow along the pathways into your body. This is typically an unconscious process; however, if your thoughts are toxic (and we all know what that means!), that is the perfect breeding ground for disease and distress.

Your emotions, as well as negative and positive thinking, direct your qi along the meridians in your body, like water flowing downstream. Negative thinking, poor lifestyle choices, and a lack of coping mechanisms lead to a compromised and weakened immune system, which can make anyone susceptible to sickness. Lifestyle choices include the foods we eat, the exercise we get or don't get, the amount of alcohol or drugs (prescription or recreational) we use, the amount of sleep we get, and the ways we take care of ourselves emotionally.

Thoughts Are Magnets

Your thoughts work as large magnets; what you are thinking you will attract energetically. What you say and how you say it are other forms of conscious powerful attraction. As you experience natural positive electromagnetic energy, you will find it becoming easier to visualize yourself achieving what you want in life, whether it is your ideal relationship, shape, weight, job, or fitness level.

With regular practice, you will become able to visualize yourself as a healthy, happy, glowing, and relaxed person. This is the *you* you want to see yourself as, the *you* you will create for yourself. If you are having trouble seeing yourself in this way, imagine talking to a trusted friend or caring for an animal you love very much. What would you say if he or she was not well and was obviously out of balance? What would you want for him or her? How would you find the help he or she needs to get to an ideal place of wellness?

When you come up with the answers (and you will), put your ideas into action. Start your mental chain of qi moving to change its direction. You will make your new thoughts become reality. It really is an inside job. You create wellness with your inner EnerQi.

A Diet of Positive Thinking and Speaking

Allow yourself to go on a diet of positive thinking and speaking. If a thought comes into your head that is anything but positive or empowering, send it away immediately. If it doesn't feel good to think about or say, the chances are that it is not good for you or anyone else.

Learn to monitor your thoughts. Watch your thoughts flow into the field of your mind. Identify what kind of thoughts you are having. Are they positive and constructive or negative and destructive? Practice mind control and consciously choose only thoughts that serve you and others in a positive way. If what you are thinking does not enhance your life or the lives of others, toss those thoughts away, like a log that rushes down a river. You can choose to do this simply because you say so. It all starts in your mind.

It has been said that prayer is for asking and that meditation is for listening. Give yourself permission to spend fifteen to twenty minutes each day to quiet your mind, let go of all stress and just relax. There is a lot of information available on meditation techniques; find a style that fits you best. I have included an example of one practice in Chapter 6 for you to try.

In time, and with regular practice, you will notice that a profound sense of peace overtakes your body and mind and that a heightened creativity permeates your thoughts. Life's challenges become easier to experience. Cloudy questions yield clear answers when one is able to still the mind.

Running Without Pain

I first tried acupuncture because I am a runner and was experiencing pain in my hip. My general practitioner examined me, took X-rays, and said that he couldn't find anything wrong with me but that if it hurt, to stop running (not an option, if you know runners!). I tried chiropractic, with mixed results. After running through the pain for almost two years, I was open to trying anything but surgery or drugs.

Oriental medicine was a welcome and pleasant surprise, because I was treated as a whole person, not as a specific injury. Not only was my hip pain cured, I also noticed that with treatments and a few tweaks to my lifestyle choices, I no longer got cold sores and I avoided the fatigue that I had fought valiantly for years with caffeine. I found that I was totally chilled out after treatments and a lot less irritated by the little things and people in life. I am now hooked and know when I need to go in for my "attitude adjustment"!

—*T. A. S., twenty-nine-year-old female*

Chapter 6

Enhancing Your EnerQi with Sleep and Meditation

Too much of a good thing can be wonderful.

—Mae West

I often hear people say, "I'll sleep when I die," which is an interesting saying, because what people don't realize is that they are actually shortchanging themselves of the vital vibrations of EnerQi, making life a dull replica of what it could be. In fact, most people don't get enough sleep— seven to eight hours is the recommended daily dose. Your health and your ability to sleep restfully go hand in hand.

Studies abound about the benefits of sleep as well as meditation. Meditation is a resting state that can mimic the benefits of sleep. When you see an Oriental medical practitioner, he or she will ask you about your sleep habits and is likely to recommend that you engage in a meditation practice to promote your ability to relax. There are some changes you can make right now, including setting the scene for restful sleep and a daily meditation practice.

Your Bedroom Environment

As discussed in Chapter 1, our environment has its own EnerQi vibration. What is the energy you are picking up from your bedroom? Look around: Is your bedroom conducive to relaxation, sleep, and sexual intimacy? Are your bedroom and your life set up to provide the most beneficial sleeping experience?

Bedrooms are best when painted in a soothing shade. Colors representing passion and the colors of human flesh tones are good choices for the bedroom according to Chinese theory. If you can't control the color of the walls, choose accent pieces in shades of apricot, peach, red, pink, and orange tans, creamy light browns. (Think evening sky at sunset). Light burgundy is an option, but not too purple (since purple represents stagnation, in the Chinese system).

Ideally, face your head to the north and your feet away from the door. When you walk into your bedroom, strive for a feeling of peace and serenity to come over you, as if you have just entered a relaxing spa or a temple. If you must have a TV in your bedroom, avoid having it be the focal point of the room, or find a decorative piece of furniture to store it in. Your bedroom is where you go to rest and recover from the world; make it a reflection of your idea of a sanctuary.

Are Worries Keeping You Awake?

If you lie awake thinking and worrying, it is time to be honest about why. Are you worrying about money challenges? Do you live beyond your financial means? Is some aspect of your work unfulfilling or just no longer working for you? How are the relationships in your family? If you are with a significant other, do you feel safe and happy within that relationship? Whatever is on your mind, think about these issues outside the bedroom, so that when you prepare for bed you can let go mentally and relax. Think honestly about your concerns during the daytime. There is a saying: Worry takes happiness out of the day and sleep out of the night.

Rather than worrying endlessly, day and night, shift your thinking by reframing how you think. Make a conscious decision to strategize, looking for ideas and inspiration within your situation rather than focusing on the daunting dilemma of your challenge. Keep in mind that everything changes. Can you remember what kept you awake five years ago at 11:00 PM on a Thursday? You can choose to reframe your thoughts just because you say so. (For more on changing your thinking patterns, see Chapter 5.)

Your Key to a Good Night's Sleep

Sleep allows your body, the engine that takes you around in your life, to shut down and regenerate. People who do not schedule enough sleeping time or do not rest well when they do sleep are more prone to frequent colds, anger, moodiness, depression, forgetfulness, impatience, and indecision. Their minds are less sharp, they seem on edge, and they are often just not "with it." We have all seen examples of this type of person walking around or, worse, driving (it is not a pretty sight!). Over time, lack of sleep compromises your immune system, your thinking abilities, and your metabolism and speeds up the aging process.

Acupuncture alleviates sleep disorders, so if you have not had a treatment yet, this could be your key to a good night's sleep. If you are experiencing dream-disturbed sleep on a regular basis, it might be a sign of unresolved emotional conflict. We often emotionally process much of what goes on in our waking hours during our sleeping hours.

If this is happening to you, it might be a sign to look at your life and make some changes. It is not uncommon to awaken during the night to use the bathroom and then go back to sleep. However, if you are having trouble getting back to sleep—tossing and turning, watching minutes and hours tick away—you have a choice to continue and be frustrated and tired in the morning or to relax and meditate.

By relaxing and breathing, you can shut down the mind and allow the body to let go of all tension. Remember what was said earlier about positive thinking: If what you are thinking does not enhance your life or the lives of others, toss those thoughts away, like a log that rushes down the river. It all starts in your mind.

Quiet the Wandering Mind with Meditation

Your mind can take you anywhere you let it. It can be hard to focus on finding a quiet place inside because the mind will just not turn off. This occurrence is referred to as a *wandering or a monkey mind*. What can quiet the mind is meditation, and in doing meditation, practice makes perfect.

First, create your own relaxing happy place, inner temple or sacred space by envisioning your perfect environment. For some, it helps to imagine a scene in nature that most appeals to you: a beautiful ocean, a majestic mountain, a flowing clear stream, a cloud-filled sky, or a rolling field of flowers. If you are more kinesthetically inclined (i.e., a tactile learner), holding on to an object such as a smooth gemstone or something that holds a special meaning for you can be quite calming. In this calm place, allow yourself to be free of distractions.

Then try this simple meditative breathing exercise.

- Begin by just closing your eyes. Relax the muscles around your eyes, your jaw, and the rest of your face. Relax your belly, arms, hands, fingers, legs, feet, and toes. This feeling is akin to floating on a raft. Slightly open your jaw and relax your mouth and throat. Breathe slowly through your nose, feeling your breath begin to fill up your belly as if you were filling a large golden orb of light.

- When you have filled up your belly to the point of comfort, exhale slowly and deeply through your mouth with even and slow breaths, allowing your belly and solar plexus to flatten. Inhale again, slowly filling up with your breath, filling that golden orb of light, and then exhale deeply. Allow all this breathing action to happen in slow motion. With the inhalation, envision deep peace and serenity. With the exhalation, feel all the tension leaving your body, along with any fear, anxiety, sadness, and confusion.

- Continue this breathing cycle until you feel yourself beginning to relax from your head to your toes. You may find yourself drifting off to sleep, and that's okay. If you go back to your thoughts, allow yourself to just watch them float away like logs going down a stream. Using long and languid breaths, continue to deeply inhale and then deeply exhale. Some find that repeating a mantra or an empowering phrase in the mind's eye helps them to quiet the wandering mind. Listening to soft music or a hypnotherapy recording is another wonderful way to learn to relax and rest.

Daily meditation (from fifteen to twenty-five minutes) can be very helpful in the cultivation of a more relaxed and open approach to your daily life. There are many approaches to developing a daily or weekly meditation practice. Remember that there is no one-size-fits-all approach, so don't worry if you are doing it correctly or sitting in the right position. Just begin now, right where you are. As cloudy questions yield clear answers, one's pathway begins to unfold from a newfound space.

Think of this practice as a higher mental training that must be mastered. Remember, the mind leads the qi.

Dr. Tan once told me something I have never forgotten: "Life is an experience not unlike a huge roller-coaster ride. There are great highs and long lows, but it is how one rides that is the key to happiness."

Enjoying a Full Night's Sleep

After years of restless sleep, I was walking around exhausted, with true memory loss and impairment. My immune system was beginning to falter, and I was catching cold after cold. A friend of mine suggested I try acupuncture, and frankly, I was sick of taking nighttime sleep aids. This was not what nature intended!

As I lay there during my first treatment, I was incredibly relaxed. I actually fell asleep on the table! I hadn't slept like that in years. As soon as Sheri put the needles in, it felt like a mild form of laughing gas from the dentist. By the time she closed the door, I was floating and on my way to a deep, relaxing nap. This relaxation stayed with me throughout the rest of the day; in fact, I was actually tired the rest of the evening and slept for five hours straight after my first treatment! I hadn't done that in years.

After six months of treatments and herbal medication, I now enjoy a full night of sleep every night. It has changed my life. No more colds! I can concentrate at work and I am so much happier; just ask my husband!

—*A. L., forty-eight-year-old female*

PART III

Inform

We think in secret and
it comes to pass,
For environment is but
our looking glass.

—James Allen

Chapter 7

Empowering Relationships: The Company You Keep

If you can't find the truth right where you are, where do you expect to find it?

—Dōgen

Until you are clear about your desires and motivations in all aspects of your life, it will be impossible for the universe to give you what you need and want. I am not suggesting that you should know all the answers in this moment to any given situation or that you are less than perfect for not having answers or ideas about where you are now. However, surrounding yourself with like-minded, forward-moving, creative, healthy-thinking people who make you want to become a better human being in all ways will set the bar high for the free-flowing expression of powerful EnerQi.

Answers to life are easier to reach when you are in an empowering relationship with yourself and with others. Relationships can certainly be difficult, but they can also be incredibly rewarding, bringing all who participate in them much joy and growth in this game called life. Begin now to inform yourself about your relationships. Start paying careful attention to the people in your life and the relationships you experience with them and with yourself as a result.

The Company You Keep

When your friends win, you win. Your EnerQi becomes enhanced with the vibration of positive movement, momentum, and happiness. Your friend's vibration becomes yours; your energy plays off each other. In short, you become the company you keep.

Take a look at the people you have around you, those with whom you are the most intimate. Do their values illuminate the light you want others to see when you think of them? Do your friends lift you up to higher levels of love, happiness, spirit, creativity, and intellect, or do you need to lower your standards when you are with them? These are important questions to ask yourself.

If your relationships are holding you back rather than empowering you, consider why. Do you feel deserving of loving and empowering relationships? Do you know how to have such relationships? I have found that the best way to have the most empowering relationships with others is to make sure your relationship with yourself feels loving, comfortable, and empowering. This is achieved by living a balanced life and regularly taking steps to maintain your health and well-being. As you align yourself honestly with your goals, desires, and inner joy, people who support, respect, and understand you will show up in your life in wonderful ways.

Those who do not resonate with your EnerQi vibration will naturally fall away because of your healthy forward momentum in life. When a relationship no longer fits, you may need to have a conversation with the other person to bring the relationship to a conclusion. Such a conversation can always be done with compassion, love, and honesty. Bringing truth to light can offer both parties' relief and clarity—a gift you give to yourself and others.

As your EnerQi vibration continues to increase, you will find that you begin to attract people into your life who are on the same frequency as you. Your relationships with these people will grow naturally from a well-grounded, positive foundation.

Releasing Old Relationship Wounds

It is much easier to enjoy empowered, confident, fun, and loving relationships when you feel balanced and are in harmony with the inner wisdom that comes from strength of body, mind, and spirit. As acupuncture helps move energy freely throughout the body, it can release any stagnation (blocks) that may be interfering with the development of healthy, supportive relationships. As the electromagnetic currents created from the needles course up and down the many meridians, they take with them old, accumulated emotional debris, such as long-held negative beliefs, anger, frustration, and sadness.

Negative feelings become less prevalent. They are replaced by newfound energy, positivity, and happiness. The mind feels clearer. It becomes easier to take deep breaths and see life from a bigger, more enhanced perspective. The body, mind, and soul just work better. With regular acupuncture sessions and a health-maintenance program, many people find that their capacity increases for taking action on relationship issues and related situations that previously seemed unapproachable or overwhelming.

Engaging in a More Intimate Nature

Sexual health is of great importance in moving and maintaining healthy qi. Sex is something most adults think about, have in common, or participate in. For the greatest fulfillment in an intimate relationship, open communication, awareness, and knowledge of yourself and your needs are important components, in addition to letting go of fear, rejection, shame, embarrassment, control, and competitiveness.

When considering what you want in a sexual experience, be present with your physical, mental, and emotional self. The EnerQi you bring to your own experience will be what is brought back to you. Make the most of your happening. Show up for yourself and your partner. An orgasm will enhance your EnerQi.

When an Intimate Relationship Is No Longer Working

When we stay too long in a relationship that is no longer working, it creates stagnation both in our own lives and in the life of the other person in the relationship. A lot of people get stuck in the thought of "but I love him [or her] so much."

Here is a consideration: Lasting relationships are not always just about love. It is very helpful, perhaps imperative, to also have liking, respect, shared ideals and interests, and compatibility. You can choose to have some or all of these qualities in your relationship with another depending on what you are looking for and what is present between you. Sometimes, no matter how much we bend or compromise, we just can't create our vision of who we really are in the relationship or who the other person is to us.

Compromise in any relationship is very important; no one person will ever be able to fulfill all our desires. Seeing who another person is clearly without making him or her wrong, or creating drama for who he or she is, is very important for peace of mind and for the continued opening of your heart. If you are not connected and truly enjoying most of your time spent with your partner in the good and bad times, start honestly looking at yourself, your partner, and your motivations. It is the only way to have optimum EnerQi flow and happiness in your life.

People don't change or compromise unless they want to. All the crying, cajoling, anger, and arguing in the world won't alter that fact. You can only change yourself. Every relationship has a life-and-death cycle. The key is to allow movement and honesty in that expression.

Awakening Sexuality

I had been celibate for fifteen years and was resigned to the fact that I was going to stay single and be alone. Lo and behold, I then met a man, and we clicked! My sexual desire had been asleep for the past ten years. I was excited (excuse the pun) to resume lovemaking but found I was less able to lubricate. I did not want to use artificial hormones.

I have always been pretty fit. Sheri gave me some wonderful and relaxing treatments that calmed my nervousness and helped to get my juices going. I began to drink a nice-tasting hot herbal tea and started eating some natural hormone–producing foods. I am happy to report that life is wonderful in and out of the bedroom. Thank you, Sheri!

—*N. P., fifty-seven-year-old female*

Bye-Bye, Baby Blues

After the birth of my second son, I was looking for a natural solution to remedy the baby blues. My acupuncturist was instrumental in helping me get better, and I am so grateful. She takes the time to really listen and understand everything going on in my life and treats me based on those symptoms and factors.

It was amazing how much better I felt after my first session! I was feeling more like my normal self, I had increased energy, and the baby blues feelings had significantly decreased. After four sessions, I'm happy to say that the baby blues have completely diminished, and I'm back to my vibrant, happy, energetic self. Words can't express how thankful I am. Sheri's incredible energy, positive attitude, serene environment, and masterful talents helped me to bounce back quickly so I could truly enjoy this wonderful time with my family.

—M. P., *thirty-seven-year-old female*

Chapter 8

Overcoming Self-Sabotage and Addiction

A man is what he wills himself to be.

—Jean-Paul Sartre

Sex addiction, drug abuse, overconsumption of alcohol or food, addiction to drama or shopping, excessive gambling, and shoplifting are all risky, self-sabotaging behaviors that serve one purpose: to fill a hole inside the person who engages in them. If this is you, you understand what I mean by a hole. Fortunately, there are other ways to fill emptiness within yourself in much less destructive ways.

You can begin to make yourself whole by seeing clearly and honestly what your fears are, what those fears keep you from having, and why you choose to keep your addiction or self-sabotage active. These behaviors keep you from feeling truly safe, loved, happy, and respected—by yourself and certainly by others in your life. You can count on your depressive addictions running your life until you act on your own insights.

We all have flashes of brilliance and intuition. When a flash of intuition hits, it will become crystal clear what you need to do to stop self-sabotaging. Part of that is listening to what other people tell you about your behavior. Take their awareness seriously. Whatever your dysfunctional behaviors are, with insight you can begin to change them.

What Brought You Here?

Explore the deeper reasons that led you to this path in the first place. Why does your submerged self need to be high? Do you become safer, calmer, energized, and more expressive with the feelings that your high brings? Ask yourself, "What are the emotions and feelings that are holding me hostage here? What do I need to do for my physical and emotional well-being so that I may leave this place, create positive feeling safely, and get to higher ground? How can I get there from here?"

Stay vigilant, listen to your self-talk, and watch your patterns and choices regarding people, places, and things. When you are not fully connected with your higher EnerQi vibration, the situations you are in and the people you surround yourself with—though seeming to be different—are often just new faces or scenes that create the same scenario you have been participating in over and over again. These repeat scenarios keep you from raising your EnerQi vibration to higher levels of health and mental and emotional wellness.

Get Really Real

Within the scenarios that play out in your life, watch who you are being spiritually, physically, emotionally, and intellectually. What do you really want for yourself? Will this situation or your other choices bring you that highest intention? How is your vibration? How do you look physically? Do your inner thoughts support you? Are you having fun? Are you feeling happiness?

It is going to take tremendous honesty and insight for you to see yourself and your patterns clearly. You may have to practice hourly mindfulness in the beginning if you want to see change. Remind yourself regularly of your goals and higher aspirations. The way in is truly the way out in this case. At times like this, connecting to and using your deep EnerQi conduit can be very difficult because your power for choice can be lost in the moment of unhealthy obsession. It is often impossible to move along without someone pushing from behind. Are you ready and willing to reach out and grow?

Me Is *We* Upside Down

To change your weak vibration, you must be willing to turn your life in a new direction and change the way you view it. This change will move you onto a renewed path that leads to an empowered pulsating EnerQi field. Get yourself on the proverbial train now to begin your journey.

An important step is to forgive yourself for your detour into negative temptation. You can make amends to the people who have supported you, stuck by your side, and believed in you later in your process, as you start to feel better and resolve your unwanted conflicting behaviors.

Now is the time to throw away your old stuck ideas about who you are and begin to create a new, more powerful you. Life is about ongoing transformation; most situations, like the seasons, are temporary. Give yourself permission and the will to transform.

Put together a team of people you like, respect, and trust: a medical doctor, a therapist, an acupuncturist, a massage therapist, a chiropractor, a nutritionist, a trainer, a life coach, and an intimacy coach. Make sure to get a complete physical examination from the professionals on your team. You may be a candidate for long- or short-term pharmaceutical intervention. We are looking for an honest, integrative approach to discovering balance within you, taking into account all your particular needs.

Find a wellness group, a twelve-step program, a non-twelve-step program or a support group that you feel comfortable with and that meets regularly. Find a sponsor. Let these people hold you accountable for your goals. They will support you in standing tall until you can do so on your own, if you allow them to. As you do whatever it takes to become healthy again, you will begin to see subtle changes in your body, mind, and EnerQi: more energy, increased EnerQi vibration, improved appetite for healthy foods, renewed sleep, clearer thinking, less negative self-talk, balanced emotions, and a return to moments of happiness and laughter.

What Brings You Happiness?

Visualize yourself participating in your life without your self-sabotaging behavior.

Figure out what makes you laugh and what brings you joy. See yourself doing these things regularly. What other activities or hobbies can you see yourself doing that will bring you even more fun, joy, and relaxation? Create a vision board, or write your ideas down in a journal daily. In talking with my patients, I have come to understand that everyone has a special talent that makes him or her happy when it is put to good use. With thought and desire, you can find your special personal talent. There are personality tests readily available that can support you in finding the areas that you excel in. A career counselor also has the expertise to support and guide you.

Healthy fun and laughter generate feel-good endorphins in the mind that stabilize mood and emotions. There really exists, in this universe, another sense of peace that you can begin to carve out for yourself. Part of your personal growth journey is having the willingness to put what no longer works behind you and look ahead to what does. There is a wealth of valuable information available about who you really are and what you need to discover as you move toward change.

Use this time right now to create your silver lining; make it your defining moment. Link yourself up to your EnerQi connection. This connection will lead you to health, wholeness, and balance. The more you practice taking control of your mind, the easier it will become to consciously choose only that which serves you and others in a positive, loving, and intelligent manner. You will find that you truly experience life in a whole new way.

Acupuncture Can Help

Acupuncture is incredibly helpful when you need to make sweeping changes in your life. With the stagnation that occurs throughout many years of engaging in destructive unconscious behaviors, a good "sweeping" can assist you in letting go of what no longer serves you. Through acupuncture, and Oriental medicine in general, your EnerQi vibration can be raised to a much higher level.

Knowing What It Feels Like
to Be Balanced

When I first walked into Sheri's acupuncture clinic, I was 108 pounds in a five-foot-ten frame. So much has changed! Six months earlier, I had left a treatment facility for anorexia, but within a short time I could feel myself losing weight again. Sleep was eluding me. I was very afraid and knew I needed help.

With regular acupuncture treatments, I started to sleep again, and my anxiety level was greatly diminished. I started to see my life and myself differently. I began gaining weight and felt healthy about it. I have now gained twenty-five pounds and feel so grateful to finally be at a different place in my life. I had always wondered what people meant when they talked about being "balanced." Now I know it's not some New Age term. It is a really wonderful feeling. Acupuncture saved my life!

—*J. A., female, late twenties*

Happily Functioning

I have been a patient of Sheri's for seven years. Acupuncture, herbs, dietary modification, meditation, and the exercise regimen Sheri designed for me has changed my life. Before becoming Sheri's patient, I was a functioning alcoholic. Today, with the help of my support team, I am sober and have never been happier. I recommend acupuncture to anyone who wants to become more balanced and feel empowered to make and maintain changes in his or her life.

—R. P., forty-six-year-old male

PART IV

Natural

THE MIND IS LIKE A PARACHUTE;
IT WORKS BEST WHEN IT IS OPEN.

—*Anonymous*

Chapter 9

Understanding Acupuncture

Life belongs to the living, and he who
lives must be prepared for changes.

—Goethe

The Chinese first became aware of the principles of acupuncture more than 5,000 years ago when warriors discovered that certain physical maladies began to improve after receiving puncture wounds from sword fights. Chinese physicians began to take note of the correlations between puncture sites and improved health. They theorized that qi is the energy or life force that circulates throughout the body, carrying with it the body's blood and oxygen and ensuring the healthy functioning of all the bodily systems, organs, and cells. By puncturing the body in specific places, the physicians found they were able to stimulate the body's qi to heal itself.

President Richard Nixon is credited with bringing acupuncture to the United States as a new modality of medicine in the 1970s. James Reston, the *New York Times* reporter who was traveling with the president on his 1971 trip to China, got appendicitis, and his postoperative pain was relieved with acupuncture. Reston was so amazed by the experience that he wrote an article about it, and this was most Americans' first exposure to the practice.

It is no surprise that what is old is now new again, just as in the cycle of life. Like fashion trends that resurface, the acupuncture of today is based on a premise derived from ancient times, although it is carried out in a new way.

What the Studies Show

A series of recent studies using ultrasound found that meridians lay along sheets of connective tissue that surround the organs of the body. The scientists found that 80 percent of the acupuncture points correlated with major connective tissue planes along the meridians. They also found that acupuncture stimulates the hypothalamus and the pituitary glands, which increase the immune function and improve one's mental state. Acupuncture acts on these brain structures to control appetite, moods, drug cravings and food cravings. Doctors now routinely prescribe acupuncture for pain management and substance addictions. Acupuncture lowers levels of neurotransmitters, such as norepinephrine and dopamine, which are often elevated in people who experience stress and pain.

Chronic pain sufferers, who feel unable to break the cycle of pain, often experience clinical depression. Acupuncture helps both pain and depression by releasing endorphins and serotonin, which enhance the body's ability to heal itself. The effects of acupuncture have been shown in studies employing brain scans. The scans showed decreased activity in the limbic system, which is the area of the brain that controls emotions.

Many acupuncture patients report experiencing a deeper awareness of self and a greater capacity for enjoyment and creativity. When patients with addictive challenges are able to stabilize their emotions, they reduce the nervous and repetitive behaviors that feed what may be unfulfilled emotional needs.

The Needles and the Electromagnetic Force Field

Acupuncturists use needles and their electromagnetic properties to release, charge, and balance or convert qi, allowing the revitalized and changed life force energy to flow into the body. The needles used during an acupuncture treatment are metal and therefore conduct their own invisible electromagnetic energy field.

When we insert sterile, disposable acupuncture needles along strategic points in the body called acupoints, the meeting of the needles and the body's electromagnetic force fields balance the body's entire energy field. We add energy or qi by twirling the needles, where it may be lacking or take away excess energy or qi where it may be overstimulated. By placing the needles accurately in the body along the meridians, or energy channels, we can strengthen weaknesses, sedate excesses, warm or cool the body, or disperse stagnation to once again allow a healthy flow of energy.

Acupuncture's Increase in Popularity

Acupuncture has gained in popularity because many people believe that Western medicine does not fully address their health, weight, and wellness needs or that certain Western medicine methodologies are too invasive and carry lasting or uncomfortable side effects. These people, like you, are searching for alternatives to fill that gap. Americans are increasingly turning to acupuncture to proactively maintain their health. They are finding relief in the fastest-growing modality of health-care treatment in the United States, with more than 8.2 million Americans turning to acupuncture today.

Organizations such as the National Institutes of Health and the World Health Organization have studied acupuncture and its effects and recognize its power to treat a wide range of conditions. Evidence of its efficacy are growing with studies using brain scans and ultrasound, which demonstrate that acupuncture creates direct, measurable, positive effects on the body. For instance, a study at the University of California at Irvine using functional magnetic resonance imaging showed that the visual cortex in the brain was activated when the scientist's inserted needles along the acupoints on the foot that are responsible for vision.

Western Medicine Versus Oriental Medicine

In Western medicine, it is common to treat illness after the fact rather than promoting balance and wellness to prevent illness from occurring in the first place. Too many people wait until a disease has taken hold in their bodies, even though they know they feel off balance. Waiting risks weakening the immune system or changing the metabolism. When the immune system or the metabolism is affected, disease, weight gain, or weight loss are the result.

Many patients seek conventional medical doctors for a myriad of medical challenges but receive prescriptions to treat symptoms instead of solutions for the root cause of the health challenge. Many doctors are not aware of the benefits of acupuncture because they lack training and exposure to Oriental medicine, and they are therefore hesitant to refer patients to Oriental medical pracitioners.

In essence, Oriental medicine focuses on balance and wellness, which helps to prevent illness and lifestyle imbalances. Acupuncture also provides a boost to your body's recuperative powers and your metabolism, enabling you to recover your health quickly. You will find that acupuncture is truly a wonderful and effective medical approach that empowers your body to heal itself. You can expect to feel better while also learning what makes your body feel healthier, stronger, and more balanced.

Although acupuncture has no religious affiliation, many patients experience a deeper spiritual awareness from its profound relaxing effects on the nervous system. Along with the unique calming effects of a treatment come the ability and the desire to go deeper within. Cloudy questions become clearer, resulting in answers. Where there was once mental inability, there is newfound clarity, enhanced emotional ability, and sustained willpower.

Many people try acupuncture when they have exhausted all contemporary Western medical options. They have often been given the choice of drastic surgery, more drugs, or continued pain and suffering because nothing further can be done for them. They are desperate and ready to try something new. Many of my patients fall into the "not sick but not well" category. They fall through the cracks of Western medicine, and acupuncture can often help.

In my practice, I have successfully treated the following conditions with acupuncture:

- Body image challenges: weight gain, weight loss, obesity, anorexia, and bulimia.

- Dermatological issues: eczema, psoriasis, acne, shingles, herpes (oral and genital), hair loss, edema, and hives.

- Ears, eyes, nose, and throat conditions: infection, cold, flu, bronchitis, pneumonia, earache, sore throat, sinusitis, asthma, ringing in ear (high or low), and the beginning stages of hearing loss.

- Emotional or mental pain: panic attacks, anxiety, depression, mood disorders, attention deficit disorder, sleep disorders.

- External systems: addiction (to prescription pain medication, recreational drugs, food, or alcohol) and hangovers.

- Allergies: hay fever, seasonal, and food.

- Internal organ conditions: stomach indigestion, nausea, irritable bowel syndrome, colitis, ulcers, constipation, hypoglycemia, hemorrhoids, stroke, Bell's palsy, trigeminal neuralgia, cerebral palsy, polio, and chronic fatigue.

- Memory challenges.

- Meniere's disease and vertigo.

- Conditions of the muscles, tendons, ligaments, and nerves: fibromyalgia, arthritis, back pain (upper, middle, low), sciatica, neck pain, shoulder pain (including frozen shoulder syndrome), tendonitis, stiff neck, bursitis, carpal tunnel syndrome, temporomandibular dysfunction, and tennis elbow.

- Gynecological issues: premenstrual syndrome, amenorrhea, cramping, infertility, menopause symptoms (hot flashes, night sweats), menorrhagia (flooding), pelvic inflammatory disease, and ovarian cysts.

- Poor self-image.

- Pregnancy: infertility, morning sickness, breech presentation before delivery, inducement of labor, lactation insufficiency, and milk fever.

- Presurgical and postsurgical care.

- Seasickness and motion sickness.

- Sexual dysfunction (male and female).

- Sports injuries: sprains and strains.

- Stress: high or low blood pressure, headaches.

Animals also benefit greatly from acupuncture treatments and herbal medicine.

Although most of the above health issues do not prevent someone from living his or her day-to-day life, they can all make life more difficult than it has to be. Some of these imbalances are certainly more challenging than others. However, I have seen positive changes in all my patients regardless of the severity of their symptoms.

People who have autoimmune disorders often use acupuncture to support their immune system function. In my practice, I have also treated patients with AIDS, cancer, diabetes, hepatitis, lupus, Lyme disease, gout, multiple sclerosis, Parkinson's disease, and other serious autoimmune disorders, as well as babies with sleep challenges and failure-to-thrive symptoms.

If you are bruised, swollen, sick, inflamed, in pain, or otherwise under the weather, run, don't walk (limp if you must!) to an acupuncturist. The sooner you get yourself there, the faster you will recover. If you have never been to an acupuncturist before, the next chapter will let you know what to expect. Keep in mind, however, that your acupuncturist will guide you through the session, letting you know what to expect and when.

Regaining Strength and Finding Confidence

I first discovered acupuncture in February 1998. I was desperate. I couldn't work for six months because of extreme muscle weakness, aches, dizziness, and stiffness in my joints. I had lost fifteen pounds and couldn't gain weight, no matter what I ate. I had an erratic menstrual cycle and loose bowels. I had been to several doctors, and every test turned out negative. I had been told by a couple of doctors that I had chronic fatigue syndrome and that there was nothing they could do. I was resigned to the fact that I would probably be this way the rest of my life, because all the literature on the topic was doom and gloom.

Through a friend, I found acupuncture. I was assured that I could be helped, which was a shock to me, especially after all those months of doctors telling me nothing could be done. I was scared but decided to try it. My stiffness noticeably improved after my very first visit. My prescription was twice a week treatments of acupuncture for several months, dietary modifications, and herbal medicines. Within three months, I was back to work, albeit on a shortened schedule. It took about a year for a complete recovery.

As I continued with my treatments, I was able to look at my life differently. Not only did I regain my strength, I found a new confidence and felt more in control of my life. I am now more patient with others and myself. I have changed my diet and am healthier, mentally and physically. Acupuncture literally gave me my life back!

—*A. L. C., forty-three-year-old female*

Feeling More Alive

In December 1999, I learned I had chronic myelogenous leukemia (CML). After the initial shock and finding out that there was no acceptable donor for a bone marrow transplant, I started on a course of therapy with interferon alpha. After eighteen months of daily injections, I was depressed and extremely tired. I had also contracted peripheral neuropathy in my feet as a side effect of the medication. This condition made walking quite painful. Since stopping the medication was not an acceptable option, I had to find an alternative.

After searching the Internet and speaking with other CML patients, I learned that acupuncture might be an effective alternative treatment for the peripheral neuropathy. I was very skeptical of this therapeutic approach, since I am a doctor in the pharmaceutical field. However, out of desperation, I started on a course of acupuncture therapy.

After several months of massage and acupuncture treatments, I started to feel the pain abate. Today, I am able to walk without pain, and I feel more alive than ever. I also learned that Western medical science does not have all the answers and that acupuncture therapy should be used in a synergistic approach to the treatment of pain.

—*K. G, male, mid-sixties*

Discovering the Side Benefits

Other than experiencing a deep feeling of relaxation after each treatment, I did not realize the overall feeling of well-being and several specific health benefits until I received regular acupuncture treatments: better moods, less physical discomfort in my lower back, absence of sweating during the night, and more energy. Today, I'm high on life.

—*G. S., seventy-year-old male*

Chapter 10

Experiencing Your First Session

To be successful, the first thing to do is fall in love with your work.

—Sister Mary Lauretta

The first impression of acupuncture, like anything else, is important, and it begins as soon as the patient walks up the path to the clinic. In my experience, people show up in one of three modes: warrior, prisoner, or art-of-war. Warriors are the classic type A personality who have difficulty relaxing and shutting down their minds. Prisoners act the victim and are often very weary and afraid. The art-of-war person is more evenly balanced and is a strategic thinker, able to handle the challenges encountered in life easier than most. Which are you?

Diagnosis begins the moment you meet your practitioner and shake hands. When my eyes meet yours upon your introduction as my patient, a list of questions begins to form in my mind, such as the following: What is the shade of the whites of your eyes? How clear are they? Are your irises clear and shiny or cloudy and dull? Is your grip strong or limp like a dead fish? Are your hands clammy or dry? Do you have a distinct odor? Is it sweet, acrid, or greasy? Does your skin look appropriate for your age? Is it dewy and glowing or dry, hanging, and excessively wrinkled?

People will often be wearing the colors of their diagnosis in the clothing choices they make. In addition, the physical characteristics of the face help determine what type of personality traits you carry with you in the world. The shape of your ears and nostrils are clues to your general qi strength. The answers to these diagnostic observational questions are indicators of the general yin and yang balance in the body and are an important starting point in determining your course of treatment.

Comfortable and Confident Communication

There is a Buddhist saying, "If you can't find the truth right where you are, where do you expect to find it?" It is very important to feel comfortable, confident, and safe with your choice of practitioner. Acupuncture is a wholistic approach to health. This means that we will want to explore together, through a meaningful conversation during the intake period, who you are mentally, spiritually, and physically, and how you approach your life. This discovery is the essence of mind-body medicine.

Since all of us have different ways of communicating, it is important that you feel comfortable with your practitioner's communication style. If for any reason you are uncomfortable or find yourself not honestly sharing what really goes on in your life, certainly after several sessions, you may need to consider working with someone else. Your energy vibration must fit and feel comfortable with that of your practitioner's. If you can't be honest in what you are experiencing, or are not willing to at least explore what that is, then you are not well matched with your practitioner, or you might not be ready for help.

Your communication style says a lot about you, as do your posture and appearance. How engaged are you when answering questions? Do you know what it is you need to become more fulfilled? I will be asking myself, in this portion of the diagnosis, "Who is this person, really?" and "What makes him or her tick?" A picture is starting to develop for me.

Most people really do know their bodies; they know what is working and what is not working for them in their lives—but freely admitting it is another thing. Talking through symptoms and challenges usually helps people focus on getting in touch with what is not working and what they need. We work as partners by combining your intimate knowledge of you with my insights and knowledge. I need to get to know you to treat you.

The Questionnaire

As a new patient, you will be asked to fill out a very detailed questionnaire about how your body works, what injuries and illnesses you have experienced, and what medications and nutritional supplements you are currently taking. If you have weight issues, you may be asked to keep a four- to seven-day journal of all the things you eat and drink and to bring that journal to your appointment. This will give your acupuncturist a clearer idea of your habits.

Be prepared to answer a lot of questions, starting at the top of your head and working down to your toes. Your acupuncturist will want to know intimate details about your elimination—what goes in and what comes out—the tastes you crave, the temperature of the foods you eat, what you choose to eat, how much you eat, and when you eat it. There will be many other questions, including the following:

- After you eat, do you feel bloated and sleepy? Or do you easily digest your meals and feel energized after eating?

- How do you feel when you wake up? How about when you lie down to rest?

- Do you nap during the daytime?

- What time do you go to sleep at night? How well do you sleep?

- Do you toss and turn, or do you sleep like a rock?

- Do you have dreams that disturb your sleep?

- Are you generally hot or cold?

- Does your body temperature respond according to your surroundings?

- Do you sweat or shiver in your sleep?

- What, if anything, hurts? What is the quality of that pain: sharp and stabbing or deep and achy? Are your muscles generally tight and sore?

- What time of day or night do you have the most energy?

- How sexually active are you?

- Are you performing as well as you would like in the physical activities you engage in, including sex?

If you have decided to see an acupuncturist for an athletic injury, strain, or sprain, the practitioner will not focus on the comprehensive internal medical exam quite as deeply. Instead, he or she will want to get you out of pain as soon as possible by increasing the circulation of blood and oxygen to the area of the injury, which will help reduce the bruising, swelling, and inflammation. The practitioner will pay attention to the internal working of your body, but the first inclination will be to reduce pain.

Say "Ah"

After the question-and-answer period, you will be asked to stick out your tongue. Stick it all the way out! The examination of your tongue gives your acupuncturist a further glimpse into what is going on inside your body. The practitioner will be interested in the tongue's size, length, shape, various colors, and coating, the color of the coating, the location of the coating, the wetness or dryness of the coating, and any demarcation lines.

Your tongue tells, quite distinctly, what is going on inside your body; it provides a very clear reflection of your internal organs. Each organ has a delineated area that mirrors itself on the tongue's surface. The color of your tongue reflects the condition of your blood, qi, and yin organs. A normal tongue color is light red. Ideally, the tongue should look like a piece of fresh, raw meat. (If your tongue were for sale at the grocery store, would you buy it?) The shape of the tongue reflects the condition of your blood and qi, and its size mirrors the health or weakness of your blood and qi. The coating indicates the state of the yang organs, especially the stomach. A normal coating is thin and pale white.

Tap into This!

Next the practitioner will want to palpate your abdomen, which includes pressing and tapping. Since some people have boundaries about being touched, expect your practitioner to ask for permission to do this. The temperature of your body's *ming men* fire (see Chapter 1) can be felt right below the navel. The practitioner will look for this area to be warm.

You should not be experiencing any kind of pain upon palpation. Any unusual pain response to light pressure will be noted. The practitioner will also be looking at skin tone; cold, cool, hot, or warm temperature distribution; or any uncommon hardness.

On the Pulse

The next step in the examination is to feel the body's pulses. They are located on the inside of each wrist and can be found by placing three fingers (index, middle, and ring finger) very gently, one after the other, slightly below the thenar eminence (the pad of the thumb). You may notice a very light pressure as the superficial and deeper levels of the pulse qualities are located.

According to Oriental medical theory, we have twelve pulses: six yin and six yang. Energetically, the pulses represent the body's organ activity, which incorporates Western medical concepts of the organs. Beyond that, the idea of organ systems and ideas strongly differ in Oriental theory.

Organ pulses are divided into two main groups: the yin organs (inner and deeper) hold and store, and the yang organs (outer and more on the surface) transport and move. There are six pulses on the right side and six pulses on the left side. They are paired in yin-yang partnership, with each set representing one element of nature (fire, earth, metal, water, wood). Each yin-yang pair depends on the other to function as a whole. Since yin becomes yang and yang becomes yin, disharmony in one part of the element usually affects its pair. Your pulse is individual, indicates the current state of your condition, and is the key to your initial evaluation.

The fire element represents the heart (yin) and the small intestines (yang). The earth element represents the spleen (yin) and the stomach (yang). The metal element represents the lungs (yin) and the colon, or large intestine (yang). The water element represents the kidneys (yin) and the bladder (yang). The wood element represents the liver (yin) and the gallbladder (yang). (For a more detailed discussion of the elements, see Chapter 2.)

There is also a deeper principle within the pulses—one of pure yang and one of pure yin—that the practitioner will be feeling for within your pulse.

Another set of pulses, known as the *san jiao*, or "triple burner," are sought deeper within your pulse. These "burner" pulses are intermingled with the twelve pulses. They give further information about the inner workings of breathing, digestion, elimination, and the energy-consumption processes within your body. After a quick check of the pedal pulses, which are located on the inside of the ankles, to ascertain heart health, it is also common to check blood pressure, which ideally should be in the 110/75 for a more athletic individual and the 120/80 range for the less athletic individual.

Gathering More Information About You

If you have had any lab work done, as your practitioner I will want to look at the findings. I will also be interested to know what your cholesterol count is. If you are over age fifty, I'll want to know whether you've had a colonoscopy and what the results were, as well as the results of your most recent pelvic exam and mammogram for women and prostate exam for men.

If I decide that I need more information to make an accurate assessment of your condition, I will order more lab work through an independent laboratory or ask that you go through your primary care doctor to request those tests. Using all diagnostic tools along with the information that has been gathered from you, we can ascertain what your body needs to become more balanced and more powerful. At last, it will be time to enhance your EnerQi.

The Treatment Plan

As we review your potential treatment plan based on all of the information, it will be clear at that time how many treatments you will need in order to see the changes and improvements we will both be looking for. Everyone is different, and some people need more or fewer treatments than others. An estimate will depend on whether your condition is long-term or short-term and what your goals are.

Initially, a typical course of acupuncture treatments will be once or twice a week, sometimes even three times a week, for about six to twelve weeks. Again, the length of time depends on the severity of the symptoms. As your symptoms fade away, as you begin to feel in balance, and as your EnerQi vibration becomes strong and palpable, we will both know when it is time to reduce the frequency of your visits.

An initial consultation can last anywhere from an hour and a half to two hours, because this includes not only your initial evaluation but also your first acupuncture treatment. After your initial consultation, it is best to plan and schedule about an hour for your subsequent acupuncture appointments.

You should refrain from getting an acupuncture treatment if you have been drinking, are drunk, or are on recreational drugs. If you are taking pain medication for your symptoms, be sure to tell your practitioner.

What Is a Session Like?

Most acupuncture treatments take place in a private or semiprivate treatment room, which is quiet, clean, comfortable, and serene. Usually the patient lies down or relaxes in a reclining position. It is a good idea to wear loose-fitting, comfortable clothing so that the acupuncturist can access your acupoints easily. At your first treatment, ask to hold an acupuncture needle so you can become more comfortable with it. Most people are surprised by how tiny, flexible, and interesting the needles look—not at all what they had imagined them to be.

All needles are prepackaged, sterilized, single-use, and disposable. They are made from high-quality surgical stainless steel. The thickness of acupuncture needles ranges from 12 to 36 gauges, and they're half an inch to one and a half inches in length. The thinner the gauge of the needle, the less qi stimulus you will feel upon insertion.

Dr. Tan says, "The thinner the needle, the more the treatments!"

Some needles have a colored plastic handle on the top, which is usually an indication of the needle's size. Some are topped with a copper-, gold-, or silver-colored filigree head. Most acupuncture needles are like fine filaments of silver or gold. Usually they are very flexible and can bend very easily. The pointed tip is quite small yet very, very sharp. Many people think of a big hypodermic needle coming at them when they hear about acupuncture treatments, but this is not the case at all.

Some practitioners use a metal or plastic tube on the skin and insert the needles through the tube, which lightly presses down on the skin. Other practitioners (including me, for the most part) will forgo the tube and just insert the needle very quickly and precisely into the designated area of the body. The decision to use the tube method or the nontube method usually has to do with one's training, not necessarily one's skill.

A practitioner who uses a tube has studied more in the traditional Japanese or Korean methods of medicine. The qi response to the tube method is slightly reduced, as is the energetic frequency in the body. A practitioner who uses the nontube method has studied the more traditional Chinese methods. Initially, the qi insertion response is more pronounced and the energetic frequency is stronger.

The designated needling sites are cleaned before insertion with a sterile cotton ball soaked in alcohol or a fresh
alcohol swab. Upon insertion of the needle, you may feel
a pinch, or a small sting, or the sensation of a rubber band
snapping against your skin, or perhaps you'll feel nothing
at all. That is normal.

Sometimes there may be the smallest amount of discomfort for a mere moment, but it should never last for more
than a moment. Sometimes a blood vessel will inadvertently
be nicked. You may feel a bruising, aching sensation. (If
that has happened, you might get an instant bruise, which
can be treated with immediate pressure applied to the area.)
You may see a light bruise develop within hours or a few
days after your treatment.

It sometimes happens that a nerve will be touched. If that
is the case, you will feel an electric-shock sensation that
shoots up or down the area where the needle was placed.
We'll both know when that happens, and I will move the
needle immediately. These instances are somewhat common, although we try hard to avoid them. If or when they
do happen, they cause a few moments of discomfort at most.

In 3 percent of cases, someone will have what we call
needle shock. This means that you will feel faint or actually
will faint. Because most people are in a reclining position
or lying down, you won't have far to fall. You may experience a clammy, sweaty, dizzy sensation. Your practitioner
will be right there by your side, should this occur, and will

notice and remedy the situation immediately by removing the needles.

If necessary, we will revive you by putting gentle pressure or inserting a needle into one or several points on your body that are specifically for needle shock. A cool cloth, placed on the back of the neck or the top of the head, can also help. This phenomenon has happened to me twice in twenty-eight years of practice. My patients recovered immediately and went on to have wonderful sessions.

For some people, the original complaint is activated by the treatment, and you might experience a day or two of increased pain or symptoms. This is not abnormal. After that, it subsides, and you will begin to feel better. Acupuncturists are also trained in CPR and life-resuscitation techniques in case there are ever any other kind of emergencies requiring such application.

Often, after the initial prick, you may feel pressure or an aching sensation around the needle site. Some practitioners will twist the needles upon insertion, or midway through your treatment they may adjust the needles by quickly vibrating them up and down. This technique is known as calling the qi.

Sometimes there will be a raised, slightly pink or red ring around the needle insertion point, known as a histamine response. Patients often report a tingly, warm, pulling sensation as well. This is your body's qi coming up to "greet" the needle's electromagnetic field. You may feel all of these sensations or none of them, and you may even experience these sensations in parts of your body where there are no needles.

Sometimes one of the needles will buzz and then stop, and the next one will buzz and then stop, and so on down the line. Or all the needles can be activated at one time and pulsate and/or throb. All patients have their own unique qi experience as their bodies become balanced. There is no right or wrong feeling that takes place. Your experience is just that—your experience. You should never feel any extended pain that keeps you from being able to relax.

If one of the needles continues to ache, pull, or throb uncomfortably for longer than one to five minutes, alert your practitioner to adjust the needle so that you are more comfortable.

Within seconds of all the needles being placed in your body, positive changes begin to take place. You can expect to feel immediately relaxed and calm. The breath begins to slow down and flow deeper down in the chest. Usually a sigh is released from deep in the abdomen, like an "ah." We call that a confirmation sign, which means that the body is confirming that changes are beginning to take place. A stomach rumble or gurgling movement often begins, which is another confirmation sign. This is your body responding to the qi stimulus.

Usually within a few more minutes after I have inserted the needles, my patients begin to experience a very deep and peaceful relaxation, which allows for a meditative rest to emerge within your body. It is almost as if the body and mind let go of all thoughts, worries, stress, and tightness. It is not because the needling part is over. Once your body connects with the altered electromagnetic currents, this relaxation response kicks in.

Most or all negative energies are replaced with a meditative state of calmness; your body may feel light and floaty (i.e., as though you have had a couple of glasses of wine) or simply energized. Bodily tensions and pain usually subside during this time of quiet and rest, allowing the body's own ecosystem to achieve equilibrium. The streams of EnerQi within become clearer and cleaner. They have the enhanced ability to allow the body's energy, blood, and oxygen to move in a much more powerful and proficient manner.

By placing the needles accurately in the body, we can strengthen or tonify weaknesses, sedate excesses (where the body may be overstimulated), remove pain and muscular discomfort, warm or cool the body, and disperse stagnation or blocked qi.

A treatment usually lasts forty-five minutes to an hour after the needles have been placed in the body. It is likely that you will want to continue resting and choose to stay longer if space and time allow. You will feel immediately rejuvenated and ready to go about your day. Many patients report feeling incredibly relaxed the day of a treatment, and on the following days they feel revitalized and have more energy to tackle projects that they have been putting off. In the best-case scenario, body pain or discomfort has begun to subside, although for some it may take a few more treatments. Most report increased mental clarity. Cravings for unhealthy food and other inappropriate substance choices are usually reduced.

After your treatment, it is best to avoid exercise or strenuous athletics for twenty-four hours to allow the balancing that has taken place within the body to strengthen and take hold. It is also best to refrain from all forms of sexual activity, including orgasm, for the first twenty-four hours after a treatment.

Becoming a Believer

My second baby was due in two weeks. My baby was in breech presentation, and my doctor wanted to schedule a C-section. I was completely against that idea and was frantic for alternatives. I was desperate to have a normal delivery, and when a friend recommended acupuncture, I decided to give it a try. During my acupuncture treatments, I could feel the baby turning inside me. The treatments made me feel relaxed and rested. My baby boy was born in December, and although it was a hard labor, I was able to deliver vaginally. I am a believer in acupuncture now!

—*F. M., female, late thirties*

PART V

Energy

WHAT WE ARE TODAY COMES
FROM OUR THOUGHTS OF YESTERDAY,
AND OUR PRESENT THOUGHTS BUILD
OUR LIFE TOMORROW: OUR LIFE IS
THE CREATION OF OUR MIND.

—*Buddha*

Chapter 11

Becoming More Round

As we express our gratitude,
we must never forget that the highest
appreciation is not to utter words
but to live by them.

—John F. Kennedy

We each have a unique gift—a special skill, knowledge,
or deeper wisdom—that we can share with the world.
By stepping out of ourselves and into our community,
we maintain another type of balance within the world
of others and ourselves. The opportunities and ideas to
give back in a charitable manner are endless. As you give

to others, in small ways and in big ways, you will observe a shift in what you receive. Things will flow into place for you as both you and the world become more balanced between giving and receiving.

As more and more people in the world catch on, these actions will start to become more normal behaviors for us all. A domino effect will begin to occur. Your actions will cause reactions, and a veritable ripple effect through society will happen. Like the yin-yang symbol, all good deeds flow back to the source; the cycle continues.

What Does It Mean to Become More Round?

The Chinese philosophy of energy is that we operate in a constant shift or movement between yin and yang, or heaven and earth. When you look at the symbol for yin and yang, one of the first things to notice is that it is round, with two symbols enclosed within it. There are no sharp edges or angles; everything flows around in the yin and yang symbol.

Each half blends and gives way to the other. The two parts depend on each other for balance, harmony, and wholeness. Each half contains a round circle of the opposite color, representing the opposite energy within its center. Because the two parts are interdependent, they are conduits of energy for each other and within themselves. You could say they feed off each other's actions and reactions.

How does the concept of yin and yang translate into our everyday world? The decisions we make every day influence this delicate balance of our EnerQi. As I discussed earlier, everything—what we eat, how much we sleep, how active we are, and the positive or negative interactions we have with others—directly affects our EnerQi. Knowing this, we must consciously make new decisions that balance us. Some of these decisions can involve relationships within our community.

We can see the nature of balance and imbalance when we observe the circumstances that unfold within our lives based on our actions. Some may say, "We reap what we sow." Others call it karma. We may not like the messages we are getting from life when things aren't going our way. However, rather than feel indignant, take it as an opportunity to look for the message and ask, "What actions am I taking that warrant this? What seeds am I sowing, and how can I change my fate?"

Many people operate from a mindset of "What's in it for me?," which emphasizes receiving. Although it is important to take care of ourselves and those we love, we do not live in a vacuum. We are all interconnected, and our actions and decisions affect those around us. Giving to others, loved ones, our community, and even strangers serves as a counterweight to receiving and serves to balances us.

This type of giving back increases our dimension, rounds us out, and opens us up in a grander sense. It is not just about writing a check to an important cause (although that is a great way to give and is much needed in our world). This type of giving back encompasses the action of donating yourself, your time, your wisdom, and your presence to a cause or an individual.

It can be as simple as asking a store clerk how his or her day is going and waiting to hear the response while maintaining eye contact. It is holding the elevator door for someone who is running to catch it. Perhaps you can donate your time to become a big brother or big sister, read to the elderly in a nursing home, or plant trees in your community. Consciously, you step outside yourself and into someone else's world when you volunteer to help others in need.

Random acts of kindness do indeed come back to us, and they make the world a better place for us all. We have all had the experience of someone cutting us off in traffic or being rude to us in our daily lives, and the interaction stays with us for moments, hours, or even days. It affects the EnerQi of our spirit and can affect our subsequent interactions with other people, if we allow it.

Energy attracts its own type of energy; like attracts like, so be mindful of the kind of energy you are putting out there. As you embrace the principles of energy and balance within your life, you might consider participating in the concept of giving back. You will find that when you are in tune, everything seems to fall into place effortlessly.

A Year of Positive Changes

One day, I realized that my life had become all about drudgery. I was unhappy at my job, and my weight was at an all-time high. My energy was non-existent. Motivation to exercise was not a priority. Days and nights were all the same for me. I was tired, but I could not sleep. I was in a dead-end relationship with a man. And on top of all that, I had not laughed in a long time. When a neighbor recommended that I go see an acupuncturist to get rid of the doldrums, I had enough insight to give it a try.

Now, a year since my first appointment, thirty pounds of the old me are gone! I am working in a new job that I love, and I feel happy now. Life has become fun again. I look at situations differently. Exercise and energy are part of my life now, as are healthy eating, acupuncture, meditation, and restful sleep. It has been a year of positive changes, not always easy, but I can definitely say my life has really evolved for the better.

—*J. H., thirty-nine-year-old female*

Chapter 12

Embarking on Your New Beginning

Act from your inner center.
Whether things go well for you or ill, reflect:
All things must change.
Don't get elated or depressed, for nothing
in this universe will remain the same forever.
Practice even-mindedness.

—Anonymous

Balance is a powerful concept in Oriental medicine. As you've learned in the previous chapters, acupuncture serves to balance yin and yang, oxygenate your blood, enhance your energy, fuel your metabolism, and lift your mind. The delicate balance between yin and yang is affected by your daily choices: what you eat, how much you sleep, how much exercise or movement you incorporate into your day, your outlook on life, and the people and environment you surround yourself with. As you become more balanced, you will discover that it is easier to sense when you are off balance.

By tuning in to yourself and your life, you will be empowered to make stronger, healthier, and more powerful decisions. You can enhance your equilibrium. It is just a given: When your EnerQi is vibrating with a strong electromagnetic current, you will see that you attract like energies to yourself. Your thoughts are big magnets that become your reality. You will discover as you begin to live a more balanced life that you are creating and experiencing more joy, laughter, love, and happiness in all areas of your life. It is a central law of the universal energetic flow. We create with our thoughts and our energetic vibration. Consider this book a stepping-stone to creating the life you wish to lead.

All experiences—good, bad, and neutral—are stepping-stones to greater awareness and more opportunities. Stepping-stones can lead us onto a path or a walkway, through an opening, or toward a doorway. They create order and succession as they guide us toward or away from people, places, or things.

Stepping-stones are like intentions as we move toward our goal(s). In order to arrive at our destination, we must begin by taking the first step toward our vision. It is always an opportune time to consider health goals and to strategize how to achieve our goals. Each new day offers another opportunity to create a more fulfilling and healthier life, starting with diet, exercise, and a balanced emotional outlook. Creating a plan of action, then putting that new action into use, will lead your body to a positive reaction.

Devise a daily meditation plan and make a commitment to positive thinking. Now that you are familiar with all the benefits of Oriental medicine, perhaps you will adopt a regular acupuncture, nutritional, and herbal approach to your lifestyle. Just as your car has to go into the shop for regular tune-ups, your body needs regular maintenance to stay tuned and resilient!

A daily exercise and stretching practice is another vital stepping-stone to ongoing wellness. Find ways to work out that you enjoy, and integrate variety into your workouts. On sunny days, be sure to get outside and enjoy the sunshine. Take long, slow, deep, cleansing breaths. Adopt a regular meditation practice. Suffuse your mind with positive, affirmative thoughts. Have fun, make sure you are laughing, and enjoying your life!

Be sure to fill your diet with an array of seasonal vegetables and fruits. Make a point of getting enough water daily, and limit your caffeine consumption. You may not always eat perfectly, but healthier choices reflect a new respect for your goals as you walk toward wellness and equilibrium.

Walking down a different path may feel uncomfortable or foreign at first because it is new to you.

Keep an open mind as you adopt the principles of the LAINE system: Learn, Align, and Inform your Natural EnerQi. You will become recharged by newfound health and vitality.

How to Maintain Joyful EnerQi

1. **Make time daily to meditate.** There is no one right way to meditate— ten to fifteen minutes, one to two times a day, sitting up, lying down, reclining. Be present with where you are, in the moment, and then just let go with your breathing. As you learn to release attachment to mental activity, your body will begin to relax into the here and now, taking you deeper with your breath into the gap between thoughts, where questions and answers become clear.

2. **Exercise regularly.** It makes no difference what the weather conditions are.

3. **Stay in touch with your healthy sexuality.** Keep it alive—use it or lose it.

4. **Eat a balanced diet.** Include plenty of fresh seasonal organic fruits and vegetables. Be sure to drink enough water throughout the day. Avoid too much caffeine, sugar, and alcohol.

5. **Live in integrity.** Be your word; do what you say you will do when you say you will do it. Tell the truth; talk in ways that make others want to listen.

6. **Make your surroundings a reflection of your creative self.** Keep your home and office space neat; decorate with care.

7. **Let go of what you no longer need.** Get rid of things, old stored-up anger, relationships that no longer work, and activities that no longer serve you. Redecorate your home, move things around.

8. **Simplify your life.** Allow yourself to say no to constant activity.

9. **Remember that all things change.** Nothing in life ever stays the same.

10. **Embrace the life you have created.** Play, make time to enjoy pleasurable and interesting things, listen to music, dance, laugh, spend time outdoors, and have fun.

11. **Help others.** Volunteer when you can, and give to those who are less fortunate.

12. **Trust your higher self.** Listen to and honor your intuition.

13. **Give thanks and live in gratitude.** The more we say thank you, the more we find to be thankful for.

14. **Allow love into your life.** Feel it, give it away, and strive to always surround yourself with loving thoughts, feelings, people, and actions.

15. **Smile and savor these moments.** Life is best lived by forgetting the past and not fretting about what's to come.

Surround yourself with like-minded people whenever possible. We all carry with us our own EnerQi vibration; be sure yours is surrounded with positive EnerQi. And last but not least, make sure your life is filled with laughter and happiness!

Life abounds with possibility and is full of a myriad of choices from one moment to the next. You have the unique opportunity and privilege to choose the life you want to lead and the power to make the decisions that will take you to those places. With that power comes the ability to make educated choices that honor and support your body.

Welcome to your new beginning.

Namaste.

Appendix:
So You Want to Be
an Acupuncturist?

Licensed acupuncturists complete an extremely rigorous, comprehensive study program that requires approximately four years, with a full-time commitment after receiving an associate degree. Requirements vary from state to state, so check with your local medical examining board for exact regulations. In addition to learning all Western medical sciences, acupuncturists are trained in the traditional Chinese medical sciences, Chinese medical theory, Chinese anatomy (meridian and acupuncture point locations), Chinese philosophical studies, herbal medicine theory and preparation, clinical counseling, and *tui nui* (pronounced "twee naw"), which is a particular Chinese method of massage and bone setting. We must also participate for two years in tai chi and *qigong* exercise classes, which cultivate self-awareness and strengthen qi within the body. A lot of this information is presented in Chinese as well as in English.

During the first semester, you will find out if this work is your calling, because it is a challenging and all-consuming path. Many students leave after starting their second semester. The dedication to study, the constant memorization, the never-ending multiple exams, and the time requirements are enormous, humbling, and life changing.

After the second year and until graduation two years later, students are required to begin treating patients under close supervision in the community clinic or in the local teaching hospitals, working side by side with other medical and acupuncture students.

An acupuncturist's duty as a doctor is to focus, watch, and carefully observe a patient's general presentation, coloring, demeanor, gait, and posture. The whole being is taken into account, and in this way the whole being can be restored to health. A practitioner who can help restore an individual's overall health instead of just relieving the symptoms has an important place in our Western society. If this is the path that is calling to you, I commend you and wish you and your patients great success and joy along the way.

About the Author

Sheri Laine, LAc, diplomate of acupuncture, has been in private clinical practice for more than twenty-eight years. After her undergraduate studies in psychology and early childhood education, she earned degrees in Oriental medicine, herbology, and traditional Chinese medicine at the Pacific College of Oriental Medicine.

Her private practice focuses on integrative lifestyle medicine, with an emphasis on supporting individuals, athletes, and families to create balance, fitness, and happiness through healthy choices, Oriental medicine, homeopathy, herbology, nutrition, meditation, and cognitive awareness.

A sought-after speaker, Laine lectures nationally on integrative health care, creating equilibrium in one's life, women's issues, aging, meditation and addiction. This is her second book. Her articles have appeared in local newspapers, *Counselor* magazine and *Recovery View*. She can often be found running, walking, or bicycle riding in the early morning mist along the coast of San Diego or Santa Monica, California, accompanied by her canine companion, Pearl, and her loving partner, Gary.

Visit her website, *www.BalancedEnerQi.com.*